Betty Bumpers

Betty Bumpers

Champion of Childhood Immunization and Peace

Edited by Anna L. Eblen
and Martha Jane Eblen

ROWMAN & LITTLEFIELD PUBLISHERS, INC.
Lanham • Boulder • New York • Toronto • Plymouth, UK

Published by Rowman & Littlefield Publishers, Inc.
A wholly owned subsidiary of The Rowman & Littlefield Publishing Group, Inc.
4501 Forbes Boulevard, Suite 200, Lanham, Maryland 20706
www.rowman.com

10 Thornbury Road, Plymouth PL6 7PP, United Kingdom

British Library Cataloguing in Publication Information Available

Library of Congress Cataloging-in-Publication Data

Betty Bumpers : champion of childhood immunization and peace / edited by Anna L. Eblen and Martha Jane Eblen.
pages cm
Includes bibliographical references and index.
ISBN 978-1-4422-2127-7 (cloth : alk. paper)—ISBN 978-1-4422-2128-4 (electronic) 1. Bumpers, Betty. 2. Immunization of children—Government policy—United States. 3. Vaccination of children—United States. 4. Health promotion—United States. 5. Centers for Disease Control and Prevention (U.S.) I. Eblen, Anna L., 1947– II. Eblen, Martha Jane.
RJ240.B48 2013
614.4'7083—dc23
2013015708

∞™ The paper used in this publication meets the minimum requirements of American National Standard for Information Sciences Permanence of Paper for Printed Library Materials, ANSI/NISO Z39.48-1992.

Printed in the United States of America

This book is for the newest great generation, especially
Eblen sisters' grandchildren:
Laela, Evan, Max, Emma, Juliet, Evie, Owen
and
Bumpers grandchildren:
Emily, Callan, Meg, Alex, Linn, Braeden, Will

Contents

Acknowledgments ix
Editors' Preface xi
Anna L. Eblen and Martha Jane "Jennie" Eblen

I: Advocacy

1 Coming Together for a Better World 3
Anna L. Eblen and Colleen Kelley
2 Networking for Children's Health 13
3 Linking for Peace 27

II: Developing as an Activist

4 Family and Neighbors Survive the Great Depression 55
5 Community on the Eve of World War II 77
6 Marrying, Creating a Family, and Volunteering 91
7 Joining Political Life as First Lady of Arkansas 105
8 Living on the D.C. Beltway 121
9 Detaching, Returning to Arkansas, and the Future 143
10 Understanding a Life Story 161
Anna L. Eblen and Colleen Kelley

Bibliography 173
Index 177
About the Editors and the Contributors 183

Acknowledgments

In addition to original interviews, we have included archived materials. Our appreciation goes to all those who gave interviews. We thank and commend the University of Arkansas Libraries Peace Links (MC 907, 907a, and 907b) and Betty Bumpers Early Childhood Immunization (MC 1204) Special Collections. The Special Collections librarians, especially Geoffery Stark, proved helpful and the materials abundant.

Thank you to Carolyn Dale for her editing expertise and support. We are grateful to readers Cheryl Malone and Bobbie Eblen for their thoughts on the early manuscript. We also appreciate the work of Marissa Parks and Robert Hayunga at Rowman & Littlefield, and we thank reviewers who offered suggestions for revisions.

Thanks go to the staff, students, and faculty of Western Washington University's Department of Communication for their encouragement and practical assistance for advising, teaching, and administrative backup as well as transcribing and editing help. We offer special gratitude to Ann Reynolds, Michael Karlberg, Gail Grafwallner, Penny Page, Margie Hovde, and Alexis Tahiri. Appreciation also goes to Lori Wisdom-Whitley and students Ashley, Tiffany, Stephanie, Stephen, Cassandra, Beth, Ryan, Jessica, and Roy for assistance with transcription, proofreading, and media. Western Washington University provided internal research grants and professional leaves that facilitated this effort. I also appreciate the support of the College of Humanities and Social Sciences and Dean Brent Carbajal.

Special thanks to Rick for his dedication to keeping computer issues under control and for his loving care always.

Editors' Preface

Anna L. Eblen and Martha Jane "Jennie" Eblen

In August 2005, more than thirty-five years after Betty Bumpers entered public life as First Lady of Arkansas, we met her for interviews about Peace Links, an organization she founded in the 1980s. We had some experience of her activism in that Jennie had coordinated the North Carolina Peace Links for years and Anna had coedited *Women Who Speak for Peace*, a book that included analysis of Bumpers's peace speeches.

We made arrangements for interviews in Bethesda, Maryland. In addition to hours of interviews, Bumpers invited us to a conference, met us for lunch, and held a dinner at her home to introduce us to influential women who were former Peace Links. Toward the end of our time together, she invited us to attend her induction into the National Women's Hall of Fame the following October. Our book was born from the heady experience at the award ceremonies and our conviction that Bumpers's story deserved a wider audience.

Not only did she accomplish a great deal in her peace, health, and justice activism, but her dynamic story has spanned almost a century—from a childhood in the rural Arkansas Dust Bowl to adulthood in the D.C. Beltway's halls of power to elder years back in Little Rock, Arkansas. The story included grassroots organizing with ordinary citizens and travels around the globe among well-known political leaders. Her gift for storytelling was evident in the interviews we conducted, and we were already familiar with her lively speeches and writing.

This book is based on her words, primarily on conversations from the interviews in Bethesda and later in Little Rock. Conversational style is spontaneous, casual, and often nonlinear. We have sought to preserve Bumpers's informal and likable manner of speaking. Along with her interviews, we occasionally incorporate her speeches and essays, particularly in the "Conversations with Betty" sections of the advocacy chapters (chapters 2 and 3). Because Betty Bumpers advocated through linking with others, we invited her associates to comment about her work in the "Connections" pages that follow her first-person accounts.

Our book is a life story yet not strictly an oral history. We selected and edited Bumpers's interviews for chronology, meaning, and readability, with the intention of preserving her unique voice. Lightly edited segments (verbs revised to past tense) from her speeches and writing are interwoven with interview materials to help capture the details of her work. In interview materials, we condensed similar stories, regularized verb tenses, and added dates, names, or explanatory notes for clarity. Overall, we followed the philosophy of historian Carson, a Martin Luther King Jr. scholar who wrote, "Autobiographical editing succeeds when the resulting narrative convinces readers that it accurately represents the thoughts of the subject."[1]

Our academic backgrounds in communication and anthropology have guided our selection of Betty Bumpers's words, our questions about her influence, and our analysis. At the same time, we realize that Betty speaks best for herself. May you enjoy reading as much as we enjoyed collecting these stories.

NOTE

1. Clayborne Carson, ed., *The Autobiography of Martin Luther King, Jr.* (New York: Warner Books, 1998), ix.

I

Advocacy

ONE

Coming Together for a Better World

Anna L. Eblen and Colleen Kelley

> I could begin fulfilling the task I had been taught was an *absolute*, and that was to leave the world better than it was when I entered it.[1]

EXTRAORDINARY ACCOMPLISHMENTS

The National Women's Hall of Fame inducted Betty Flanagan Bumpers, activist for peace, children's health, and women's leadership, in Seneca Falls, New York, in October 2005. At the induction, Bumpers received a standing ovation for her thoughtful speech about the challenges facing our global community. On that day, Betty Bumpers accepted an award that recognizes illustrious women who influence the well-being of the United States and world communities. She shared the honor with nine other women, including cultural icons Hillary Clinton and Maya Lin, architect at age twenty-one of the Washington, D.C., Vietnam Veterans Memorial.

Bumpers has dedicated more than four decades to social activism leading to this well-deserved honor. In 1991, she and former First Lady Rosalynn Carter established Every Child By Two (ECBT), a national immunization education program that extended their decades of previous immunization work. ECBT evolved from a multiagency immunization effort that Betty Bumpers brought together when she was First Lady of Arkansas. Carter and Bumpers worked with a network of heath care agencies to stop preventable childhood disease. During the years when unwarranted controversy swirled around childhood immunizations, Bumpers remained committed to children's health. She organized and spoke on behalf of ECBT, confident as continued scientific evidence vindicated immunization safety. The National Institutes of Health named a new facility the Dale and Betty Bumpers Vaccine Research Center to honor the Bumperses.

Betty Bumpers also founded Peace Links: Women Against Nuclear War, an organization dedicated to grassroots peace education and women's leadership. While nuclear proliferation threatened the safety of the planet, Peace Links managed a high-profile, nonpartisan peace education program. Bumpers activated a women's network that helped publicize nuclear freeze concepts. Her interviews popularized a family-centered antinuclear stance in national magazines such as *McCall's*, *Ladies' Home Journal*, and *Parade*. Her energetic travel and advocacy produced countless articles in local and regional newspapers. During and after the Cold War, Peace Links developed global connections and leadership training for American and international women who have gone on to lead community organizing around the world.

In this book, we explore the details and significance of Bumpers's work. Our goal for the book is to give readers an account that highlights her major role in contemporary activism and that simultaneously recognizes her unique voice and stories.

Bumpers's extraordinary accomplishments grew from her roots in rural Arkansas. She and her husband Dale partnered for social change with her activism alongside his political career. An admirer of the New Deal and the Roosevelts, Betty Bumpers emulated their progressive stance as she pioneered advocacy on controversial issues, sustaining an era of increasing public participation among political spouses. In particular, she blazed a trail for future women leaders like Hillary Clinton, whose formative political experiences as First Lady of Arkansas followed shortly after Bumpers's very active tenure in that position. Early in her career, Bumpers recognized the potential of networking as an advocacy strategy effective in implementing change. She succeeded with a remarkable combination of energy, communication, and commitment. Many women now hold high-profile positions and lead communities with skills that they developed in Peace Links, ECBT, and other social change efforts that Bumpers championed. From lessons learned in her Depression-era rural Arkansas community to successful advocacy networks, Betty Bumpers's colorful personal stories show how women lead peace, health, and social justice progress.

In her elder years, Bumpers has continued to advocate for social justice. A recent article in an Arkansas magazine stated in an issue dedicated to notable regional women that "bold and resourceful, the 87-year-old powerhouse is renowned for establishing programs to immunize the nation's schoolchildren and for creating Peace Links."[2]

SOCIAL CONTEXT IN A LIFE STORY

Betty Bumpers's life story has spanned nearly a century and has interconnected with transformations in Arkansas and U.S. culture, particularly through the social movements that formed perceptions and policies about human rights, public health, and peace. Betty Flanagan Bumpers was born just before the Great Depression and near the edge of the Dust Bowl. These economic and climatic catastrophes shaped her community just as World War II and its aftermath molded her generation as they approached adulthood in the midst of unprecedented upheaval and strife. Her "Greatest Generation"[3] has faced difficult social conditions and rapid change, especially in their formative years.

The Arkansas River bisects Franklin County, where Betty Bumpers was born. With farmland to the south of the river and hills of the Ozarks to the north, the area remained mostly agricultural during recent history. Several factors came together to create a dire situation for many Franklin County families during the Great Depression. Not only did the region experience the consequences of the national financial upheaval, but also ongoing drought, depletion of natural resources, and political factors exacerbated the problems. Although not as catastrophic in Franklin County as farther west, the weather problems affected farming and migration patterns. Cotton, one of the primary cash crops of the region, both contributed to and suffered from the blowing dust. In northern Franklin County, vineyards that had experienced growth in wine production lost their market with the onset of Prohibition. Coal mining played a part in Franklin County's economy until the 1930s, and then it declined. It was only later, around the time of World War II, that natural gas, oil, and coal resources became more important again. These mixed blows led to widespread poverty, and many families struggled to make a living.[4]

To some extent, farmers who owned their land were able to provide food for their families through gardening and raising livestock, but cash was hard to come by. Schools, hospitals, and infrastructure suffered. Even when prewar defense industries began to move to Arkansas, local people were displaced, basic human services floundered, and poor infrastructure caused many problems. In the war years, Franklin County began to restore and increase its economic base; locals as well as newcomers could more easily get jobs with Camp Chaffee nearby. Jobs became available, but schools and hospitals could not keep up with the population growth, police and firefighter service was overwhelmed, and housing was impossible to find.[5]

SOCIAL TRENDS AND SOCIAL CHANGE

The young men drafted into military service traveled and met culturally different people for the first time. In Arkansas, like many other states, the war years boosted emerging social trends, such as widespread employment of women in the war industry and mass migrations of rural people, especially African Americans, to the cities for jobs and better living conditions.[6] Women and minorities lost some of these advances when the war was over. A traditional and more conservative narrative about gender and race reemerged in popular culture.

Most who had served in the military returned to civilian life after World War II. According to popular culture narrative, women happily returned to homemaking, and GIs contentedly went to college and took jobs. In the optimistic versions of the tale, couples established large families amid a stable and growing socioeconomic base. In fact, many couples, including Dale Bumpers and Betty Flanagan, did actualize this cultural narrative, although it was never as simple as the popular press proposed. Complexities arose as couples such as the Bumperses faced family problems, decided on their career paths, and dealt with the realities of child rearing. Luckily, the Bumperses settled back in Charleston soon, and their home territory ultimately satisfied positive economic hopes. In northwestern Arkansas, new agricultural businesses, such as poultry farming, began, and older ones, such as wine making,[7] became more prosperous. Public discourse of the 1940s and 1950s buttressed social cohesion and emphasized traditional roles and values, often disregarding suppressed human rights issues.[8]

As their family grew up, the Bumperses entered politics and served Arkansas from 1970 to 1999, first as governor and First Lady and then as U.S. senator and activist Senate wife. Betty Bumpers repeatedly acknowledges the significance of political position in her life: "I used who I was shamelessly."[9] Within the larger frame of women's rights and women in social movements, Betty Bumpers participated as a member of a relatively small group of women who were U.S. political spouses. Scholars propose that a U.S. First Lady's public performance is empowered and constrained by society's gender expectations about her role. These findings inform our understanding of Betty Bumpers as Arkansas First Lady and U.S. congressional spouse. Values, ideologies, political institutions, and histories of other political wives structure such women's public participation.[10]

Overall, analysts suggest that we regard political couples as a "two-person career."[11] Even before First Ladies began to speak regularly in public during the early twentieth century, presidential spouses performed political persuasion in more private spaces, such as parlor discussions, dinners, or receptions. Political wives advised their husbands and worked to enhance the public image of their spouses. The women's role evolved to include volunteerism, especially with issues that affected children and women. As models of citizenship and "a visible voice for women,"[12] some political wives pushed women's issues onto the national stage. Others went further than volunteerism and nonprofit advocacy and personally sought legislative solutions, although that path often brought censure. Critics were more likely to disparage spouses acting in the policy realm, although such innovators opened opportunities for other political wives. In the role of Arkansas First Lady, Betty had a strong public presence. She directed one of her first advocacy efforts toward public health and children's immunizations, and this effort ultimately became policy activism.

Some of the issues in U.S. public health policy had been reflected in the problems that Arkansas had experienced during World War II. At that time, the federal government intervened to provide at least two services for Arkansans and others. Roosevelt's New Deal established a rural medical assistance program through a Farm Security Administration in 1941. County associations administered localized health care, and the state board of health administered prenatal and first-year health care for military wives and infants. The medical establishment, in the form of the Arkansas Medical Association, moved quickly to thwart this "socialized medicine," but many doctors participated anyway.[13]

Nationally, public health movements had begun during the nineteenth century with discoveries about microbes and sanitation that led to groups organizing around disease prevention by the early 1900s. The success of immunization for smallpox by Jenner led to research on other diseases, with additional success in vaccines for typhoid fever and diphtheria in the early twentieth century. Through mid-century, disease prevention by vaccine became possible for other child killers such as polio, as well as rubella, measles, mumps, and other childhood illnesses that led to severe discomfort and possible disability.[14] As a part of the public health movement, Betty Bumpers's childhood immunization programs aligned governmental and nongovernmental organizations to promote early childhood immunization. While the public health movement grew and diversified in its efforts to promote general health and prevent disease, other social movements dealt with oppression related to race and gender relations.

One of the earliest significant social movements of the 1960s and particularly important in the politics of Arkansas, the modern civil rights movement grew after the U.S. Supreme Court's 1954 *Brown v. Board of Education* decision. Charleston integrated its public schools quickly and quietly soon after the 1954 Supreme Court decision. This achievement received little publicity, especially compared to the notorious 1957 segregationist dramatics of Orval Faubus in the Little Rock public schools. Dale Bumpers chronicled the Charleston events, including his work with the Charleston School Board, in his memoir. Bumpers decided to challenge Faubus's 1970 campaign for a seventh term as Arkansas governor and went on to win the governorship that year. Later, as a U.S. senator, he sponsored legislation for Charleston High School as a National Commemorative Site for achievements in equal educational opportunity.

The U.S. women's rights movement reached one goal as women achieved the vote with the Nineteenth Amendment in 1920. In Arkansas, women's suffrage groups had been active from 1888 on; they sought a state constitutional right to vote. With changes to the state constitution, Arkansas women voted in primaries after 1917, with full suffrage in 1918.[15] After slow gains through mid-century, women marked progress with more options in the public sphere. For example, voting brought women more political clout, emerging freedoms modified gender norms in the 1920s, and employment during World War II gave women a sense of their capabilities outside the home.

During the 1960s, awareness of human rights movements and, in some cases, experiences within the civil rights movement furthered women's determination to seek new goals. Many joined the "women's liberation" movement through group consciousness-raising sessions that encouraged in-depth examination of "feminine" cultural norms and behavior. Some women went on to participate in large-scale protests about equal employment opportunity, reproductive rights, and the proposed Equal Rights Amendment. In the Arkansas governor's office, the Bumperses supported ratification of the amendment,[16] but Arkansas, among other states, never ratified the amendment, and it did not become law. Nevertheless, energetic local and national participation in the women's liberation movement of the late 1960s and 1970s materialized concurrently with the peace movement. Some women activists participated equally in both movements, others stressed women's rights more than peace, and some, like Betty Bumpers, emphasized peace work over feminism.

Global peace movements have generally been cyclical, reacting to the ebb and flow of wars and their aftermath. American movements have mirrored this behavior.[17] Lofland suggests that there have been four major surges of peace movement activity in the United States, one occurring around World War I, the second in the decades before the outbreak of World War II, the third during the Vietnam War, and the fourth during the nuclear freeze.[18] Women participated significantly, and their peace efforts maintained a complex relationship with the emerging women's rights movement.

Throughout the nineteenth century, women in Europe and North America simultaneously organized against war and for their own rights in the form of women's peace societies. Women's rights and peace advocacy diverged throughout the decades of the early twentieth century. This trend lingered during the early Cold War period as evidenced by "gender-integrated peace organizations" that "neither embraced feminism nor gave women many leadership roles."[19] Later, women reemerged as peace movement leaders although often within traditional cultural norms. For example, women decried nuclear testing's strontium 90 in mother's milk during the 1962 antinuclear group Women Strike for Peace. The protests during the Vietnam War by associations such as Another Mother for Peace reinforced established feminine roles.[20] By 1980, women began to lead "not-especially-feminist" antiwar movements. One exception was Helen Caldicott's mobilization of "women *as* women who seek peace" through the organization Women's Action for Nuclear Disarmament (later known as Women's Action for New Direction) and her assertion that war was attributable primarily to men's inherent masculine nature.[21]

The nuclear weapons freeze campaign began in 1979, the idea of Randy Forsberg, a defense and disarmament researcher in Cambridge, Massachusetts. She argued that American peace groups should mutually support a proposal for a U.S.–Soviet agreement to halt the testing, production, and deployment of nuclear weapons, and many endorsed her "Call to Halt the Nuclear Arms Race." A Nuclear Freeze Steering Committee developed a 1980–1984 strategic plan that called for the peace associations to gain major interest groups' endorsement, wage campaigns to convert "middle America" to embrace its agenda, and introduce the issue into mainstream American politics.[22] The freeze campaign's first national conference was in 1981, and by June of that year, an antinuclear demonstration in New York City became the largest political demonstration in American history, with nearly a million participants.[23] After continued nuclear freeze successes, among other political pressures, the Reagan administration dropped plans to deploy the neutron bomb and agreed to abide by the provisions of the never-ratified SALT II (Strategic Arms Limitation Treaty).

Emerging in 1982, Betty Bumpers's Peace Links is situated within the nuclear freeze, the fourth major American "peace mobilization," which developed in opposition to the nuclear proliferation and foreign policies of the Reagan administration. At the nuclear freeze peak, the number of groups was nearly 8,000. However, there were fewer than fifty national organizations, most "peace associations" being "overwhelmingly local and freestanding in character." Only a few national organizations had large memberships, while many local and regional groups had smaller memberships, with twenty or fewer people.[24] Peace Links had a national organization with affiliated regional groups. Theorists continue to debate the influence of citizen activism on U.S. policy and the end of the Cold War.

Peace activism, however, became an integral part of many participants' lives. The transitory nature of many nuclear freeze organizations belied their ongoing effect on the lives of those who were members. Similarly, an immunization program may have provided a quick event with vaccines for children, but effects persisted with the lifesaving outcomes. Activists who have wanted to make the world a better place may have worked for a specific issue, but the relationships they built and the organizing skills they learned persisted. Betty Bumpers, along with like-minded leaders and role models, inspired new generations of activists who continue to shape communities.

LEARNING FROM BUMPERS'S ADVOCACY

In order to understand long-term implications of Bumpers's advocacy, we will consider the following questions:

- How does Betty Bumpers perceive the influences of people and events?
- How do language patterns in her stories reveal the meanings that Bumpers finds in her life?
- How can we better understand the lives of women by understanding Bumpers's experiences growing up and as First Lady of Arkansas and a senator's wife?
- How should we evaluate Bumpers's main contributions to society?

Our responses will arise from Bumpers's speeches, writing, and stories as she chronicles her advocacy and achievements along with the complexities and joys of her life story. In her own words, in conversations recalling events, Bumpers tells about how she became aware of social issues, why she got involved, how she approached the problems, and how she addressed the issues. Her colleagues and other observers reveal their "Connections" in essays or interviews related to Bumpers's work. By providing background and questions along with the first-person accounts, we hope to encourage readers to consider their own conclusions and insights as well.

NOTES

1. Betty Bumpers, "Remarks," 2005 Induction, National Women's Hall of Fame, Seneca Falls, New York, Peace Links Records Addendum (unprocessed), Special Collections, University of Arkansas Libraries, Fayetteville.
2. Karen Martin, "Portrait of a Power Woman," *Soiree* 4 (2012): 24.
3. Tom Brokaw, *The Greatest Generation* (New York: Random House, 1998); Neil Howe and William Strauss, *Generations: The History of America's Future 1584–2069* (New York: William Morrow, 1991).
4. "Franklin County," http://encyclopediaofarkansas.net/encyclopedia/entry-detail.aspx?entryID=410 (accessed July 15, 2012).
5. C. Calvin Smith, *War and Wartime Changes: The Transformation of Arkansas 1940–1945* (Fayetteville: University of Arkansas Press, 1986), 19–41.
6. Smith, *War and Wartime Changes*, 127.
7. "History," www.wiederkehrwines.com/history.html (accessed July 31, 2012); "About Us," www.postfamilie.com/about_us.htm (accessed July 31, 2012).

8. Cathy Collins, *America's Women: 400 Years of Dolls, Drudges, Helpmates, and Heroines* (New York: HarperCollins, 2003), 398.
9. Betty Bumpers, interview, August 2005.
10. Shawn J. Parry-Giles and Diane M. Blair, "The Rise of the Rhetorical First Lady: Politics, Gender, Ideology, and Women's Voice, 1798–2002," *Rhetoric and Public Affairs* 5, no. 4 (Winter 2002): 565–600; *Communication and Mass Media Complete*, www.ebscohost.com/academic/communication-mass-media-completeost (accessed August 10, 2012).
11. Karlyn Kohrs Campbell, "The Rhetorical Presidency: A Two-Person Career," in *Beyond the Rhetorical Presidency*, ed. Martin J. Medhurst (College Station: Texas A&M University Press, 1996), 179–95.
12. Parry-Giles and Blair, "The Rise of the Rhetorical First Lady."
13. Smith, *War and Wartime Changes*, 124–25.
14. Centers for Disease Control, "Achievements in Public Health 1900–1999: Changes in the Public Health System," www.cdc.gov/mmwr/preview/mmwrhtml/mm4850a1.htm (accessed July 20, 2012).
15. "Cotnam History," www.arkansasties.com/Special/HistoryofWomensSuffrage.htm (accessed July 29, 2012).
16. "Women's Rights," www.ualrexhibits.org/bumpers/?page_id=18 (accessed July 31, 2012).
17. "US History Encyclopedia: Peace Movements," www.answers.com/topic/peace-movement (accessed December 10, 2009).
18. John Lofland, *Polite Protestors: The American Peace Movement of the 1980s* (Syracuse, NY: Syracuse University Press, 1993).
19. Joshua Goldstein, *War and Gender: How Gender Shapes the War System and Vice Versa* (West Nyack, NY: Cambridge University Press, 2001), 327.
20. Goldstein, *War and Gender*, 327–28.
21. "Arkansas WAND News," from www.wand.org (accessed May 2, 2010).
22. Lawrence Wittner, "Mass U.S. Peace Organizations since 1957: SANE, the Freeze, and Peace Action" (paper presented at the International Peace Research Association Global Conference, Leuven, Belgium, July 16, 2008), 12.
23. Wittner, "Mass U.S. Peace Organizations since 1957," 5–6. Almost a million people rallied for a nuclear freeze in June 1982.
24. Lofland, *Polite Protesters*, 138–39.

TWO

Networking for Children's Health

> This was when I first became aware of the power I had, as a governor's wife, in mobilizing people and resources behind an issues to which I was deeply committed.[1]

CONVERSATIONS WITH BETTY[2]

"One of the most memorable days of my life was in the 1950s when my husband and I, along with hundreds of thousands of parents all over the country, marched our children down to the local clinics where they were given polio shots. I remember the air of confidence and gratitude that the people exhibited toward the medical profession in this country and the government for assuming the responsibility of helping them cope with a health problem with which they were helpless in dealing. I remember, too, as an elementary school teacher during the 50s, children coming to school early in the spring with high temperatures, rashes, runny noses, red eyes and coughs . . . the beginnings of measles epidemics, rubella or whooping cough. I also recall several cases of rubella syndrome children in my small community of 1,400 people in Charleston, and taking my fourth-grade students on a field trip to our state school for the deaf where I discovered that a very high percentage of the school's children were there because they had contracted one of the childhood diseases."[3]

"I spent the first year of Dale's governorship pondering how I could best utilize the considerable influence traditionally accorded the State's First Lady. Soon, a woman from the Centers for Disease Control called on me, and told me Arkansas's childhood immunization levels were woefully low, and asked if I would take on the task of trying to raise them."[4]

With visions of so many ill children flashing through my mind, it only took a moment to enthusiastically accept the challenge to raise the levels of immunizations against childhood disease in the state of Arkansas.[5]

"Recruiting volunteers, mostly mothers, PTAs, the National Guard, the Home Extension Economists, the Arkansas Nurses Association, and with the help of a $50,000 grant from a fund the governor controlled, we began. In our first highly publicized event, we immunized 300,000 children in one day. Soon editorial cartoonists began depicting school children jumping under their desks when they saw me coming with a huge hypodermic needle in my hand. But professionals warned me that one big splash was not a program, and that a lot of detailed work lay ahead."[6]

One of the people who helped me when I started out in Little Rock was a dear friend, Nell Balkman, a public health nurse who taught me about community organizing. We had met when Dale and I started a nursing home in Charleston in the early 1960s. I was busy with my young family at that time, so I didn't contribute to the project in a significant way. My sister Maggie's husband, Archie, became one of our partners, and although we didn't see much profit in the early years, it eventually became profitable. Following a series of rather unsuccessful attempts to better manage the facility, my sister Maggie became the administrator. She stayed on for many years in that job, and their sons still run Greenhurst Nursing Center.

When Dale and I were in the governor's mansion, I went to a workshop that Maggie hosted at the nursing home with Nell, who was president of the Arkansas chapter of the National League for Nursing. Nell traveled doing workshops for families to help adult children as they struggled when forced to switch roles with their elderly parents following admission to a nursing home. Nell assisted the families who were in the midst of working through the difficult process, and I was so impressed with the way she interacted with both the adult children and their parents throughout the workshops. She counseled those elders who had become dependent on their children to aid them in decisions about their lives. She was so intelligent and conducted the workshops with such compassion; she taught me skills that became invaluable to me in my role as First Lady.

After we'd been in the governor's mansion more than a year, a representative from the National Center for Voluntary Action (NCVA) came to see me and asked if I would help publicize and introduce the new MMR vaccine, the combination vaccine for measles, mumps, and rubella. They asked me, as First Lady of Arkansas, if I would help because of the high rate of childhood diseases against which we had preventive vaccines. We didn't have laws yet that required children to be immunized before starting school, so the NCVA and the Centers for Disease Control asked if I would help educate the people of Arkansas about the need to immunize their children. I got kind of uppity because I felt Arkansas had been tagged as the hillbilly state by Bob Burns, an Arkansas comedian and actor. And I said, "Our people don't need any more educating, but if the children need to be immunized, I'll help see to it that they get immunized."

And I added, "If you will assist me, and if you will provide the backup." They agreed, and that's how I got involved.

I immediately called Nell, and she and her staff at the Arkansas League for Nursing took me under their wing. Nell urged me to use the governor's mansion as a gathering place because people would be inspired to attend meetings in order to enter the mansion. She said, "Betty, we can do this. If you will provide the mansion as a setting, a planning place where we can gather people together to pull this off, and if you lend your name and support to it, we can do it. Work with me; we can do this."

She knew exactly what to do. First, she laid out a plan, which I could envision due to my familiarity with Agricultural Extension. Because of my childhood experience growing up on a farm, I was aware of their extensive network they had at their disposal and what wonderful work they did. I also knew that the National Guard medics could help and that a unit was available. Nell's husband was a colonel in the National Guard and stationed at Camp Robinson, near Little Rock. Dale had appointed the attorney general, who headed up the National Guard.

Nell and I contacted the American Medical Association (AMA) and asked, "If we get the children recruited and brought in, would you immunize them?"

Although Nell thought that the AMA would not agree, she wanted to involve them right from the outset so that they would not oppose our efforts. By bringing them in at the outset, they did not oppose our plans and actually encouraged their patients to come get immunizations from us. Nell convened a list of the leaders we needed, such as the head of the Arkansas Health Department, whom Dale appointed; the head nurse there; and the head of Agricultural Extension. All these department heads and volunteers rallied together to accomplish our goals. I sponsored luncheons at the mansion; being invited to the governor's mansion and being on the planning committee was really something.

We put a plan together. The head of Agricultural Extension, Runyon Deere, contacted the women who did home demonstration, and I assigned them as regional and county coordinators. We planned to use the National Guard armories for the clinics because they are located all over the state. The National Guard flew in immunization air guns and trained their corpsmen to use them. I also recruited nurses, and if we needed vaccines in one part of the state or another, I traveled. I went to every public health unit in the state at least twice during the four years Dale was governor.

"Since that time Arkansas's immunization program has become a model for the rest of the country. Since 1974 reported cases of measles in Arkansas have been nonexistent or very low. Also, within one year more than 100,000 children were given more than 400,000 immunizations, and the immunity level for polio was raised from 50 to 80 percent.

"These successes and others are due in part to the enthusiastic support of the Arkansas League for Nursing, the Arkansas State Health Department, local government officials, volunteer agencies, the Department of Education, the Agricultural Extension Division of the U.S. Department of Agriculture, the National Guard and many other interested people.

"The most effective way to implement a successful immunization program is to work in concert with local leadership . . . Dr. James E. Bowes, president of End Measles, Inc., . . . stated that the federal government can provide scientific advice and valuable assistance when called upon by the state, but the responsibility lies in the hands of state and local officials who have the authority to move the health dispensers, organize the local health officers, and conduct the clinics that get more children immunized.

"Strict enforcement of laws requiring immunization as a requirement of matriculation can be an effective means of insuring immunization of school aged children. Vaccine quality is the same whether received at a state financed clinic or by a private practicing physician. Both kinds of administration should be utilized and made available to the public. One of the things our children have a right to expect as a part of their heritage is a healthy future."[7]

I traveled to Washington, D.C.; brought the idea about having this immunization campaign; and got it established there. Pat Nixon helped me. For their administration, volunteerism was really her thing.[8] They had started a volunteer program that had a little heart as its symbol.[9] Anne Richardson, the wife of Elliott Richardson,[10] was a big part of Pat Nixon's volunteer organization and helped to put the structure for our immunizations in place. Anne flew down here, and with Nell's guidance and help, we had the plan for the immunization day all set up beforehand. We divided the state into regions, and the Agricultural Extension homemakers coordinated the local meetings. We flew in the National Guard plane or in helicopters—which was scary, sometimes—to visit all of the regions. I spent a lot of time flying with Dr. M. Joycelyn Elders;[11] she helped to coordinate "Every Child by '74" as it came together.

I pinned the Pat Nixon volunteer heart pin on the program leaders, and lots of local newspaper photos showed me or Anne Richardson—or both of us together—pinning these on. With the Agricultural Extension home demonstrators coordinating each region, we immunized several hundred thousand kids on one Saturday. That is how we pulled off that immunization in 1973. There was not one vaccine injury in that entire group of kids that one Saturday or any adverse effects from the immunizations. A lot of the kids didn't get the follow-up series of shots afterward, but a lot of them did. And even one shot was better than none.

Of course, that was just a start. Dale was not governor long enough for us to coordinate all of the county health nurses, and the structure for follow-up was not in place. That took years, and we are still working on getting follow-up for initial childhood immunizations with private doctors. President Barack Obama passed appropriations in his health care legislation that will help the private sector to computerize children's medical records. We have worked for it so long, and there is no end in sight. While immunization registries exist in nearly every state in the United States, containing vaccine histories of millions of children, they are not yet fully integrated with electronic medical records.

Immunization policy has such a long history. When we did Every Child by '74, the medical immunization effort was also working with the live-virus polio vaccine. At that time, the only indigenous cases of polio that had occurred in this country since the 1960s, I think it was, had been induced by that live-virus vaccine. The vaccine-induced polio cases were not as severe as previous polio cases, but many of them were of the paralytic type that weakened the muscles. The federal government later compensated for injuries from that live-polio vaccine. The immunization compensation bill (which Dale had a lot to do with), passed during President Jimmy Carter's administration, set up a surtax on vaccines to fund the compensations. People who have injuries that could be caused by vaccines are compensated by the federal government through the compensation fund.

Rosalynn Carter and I had become friends when our husbands were governors, and we began working to enlighten other First Ladies and enlist them in immunization work. She had heard me speak at that earlier governors' conference and had started a program in Georgia, so we already knew each other before she and Jimmy came to Washington. Later, with Dale in the Senate and President Carter in the White House, Rosalynn and I had little trouble getting money and support.

Rosalynn and I had decided to work on immunization at the national level. Rosalynn often tells the little story about how we began our partnership nationally. She says, "The first person to knock on the front door of the White House after we got there was Betty Bumpers. She wanted me to help her with the immunization program. I had already made the commitment that my first priority was mental health, and I had to follow through on that, but I did help her."

And she did. She started working with me within weeks after I went to the White House to see her. When she tells the story, I always counter by saying, "She doesn't know it, but I came to see her for two reasons. One was to see the upstairs of the White House, and the other was to recruit her to help me on this." And so the story always drew a laugh; it was a charming way to get into all of it. Two months after I went to see her, Joseph Califano, secretary of the Department of Health, Education, and Welfare, called and said, "Betty, the president tells me not to make a move on immunization until I've talked to you."

And I said, "Well, he is right. If you need to know anything about immunization or if you need any help, I'm available." We took off from there, and that was when President Carter mandated that every state meet the goal of having 78 percent of its children fully immunized by September 1978. Arkansas was the first state to meet the criteria because we had a big head start.

The Clintons were in the governor's mansion at the time, and I talked Hillary into helping me put on a reception on the grounds of the mansion, which sits on seven acres. I invited 6,000 people—I still had the list of all the volunteers from our early campaign in the counties all over the state. I sent out an invitation from Hillary and me to come to the governor's mansion for a picnic late in the afternoon on a summer day. I think it was in August, and it was a hot, hot day. I had a big surprise—I don't know how many showed up, but it was close to the 6,000 we invited. Dr. William H. Foege, head of the Centers for Disease Control, was to announce that we were the first state to meet the mandate. It was quite a celebration.

Rosalynn came to the gathering, too, and because Jimmy Carter was getting ready to run for reelection, Hillary and Bill Clinton decided to make it a big fund-raiser for the Democratic Party and the Carter campaign. They wanted to raise money and let some national fund-raisers speak. The Clintons were so interested in national politics. Dr. Foege got to give his speech and make the announcement, and the party was a great success.

With guidance from the Centers for Disease Control, Rosalynn and I visited many states while the Carters were in the White House and afterward, meeting with their legislatures and governors and all the powers that be. We wanted states to mandate that all children be vaccinated by the time they entered school because when we started, only a few states had passed such legislation. Arkansas had such a law, and Rosalynn and I went to other states and lobbied whoever would help facilitate that. Before the Carters left office, we did get all fifty states to pass laws that children entering school had to be fully vaccinated.

Jimmy Carter was defeated when he ran again in 1980, but in the meantime, Rosalynn and I had plowed right on with getting childhood immunization laws set up. Dale had taken up the bill, number 317, on the Senate floor to provide a stable funding source to the Centers for Disease Control to implement immunization programs nationwide. Dale was unflappable, even using intimidation to see that the bill passed. He'd say, "The very idea that you would not appropriate this money to take care of children!" It was a good cause to browbeat people with, and it was easy to intimidate them into voting for something like that. He kept the funding going, and we just kept pushing for it. The 317-line item of the congressional budget continues to serve as the federal funding source for immunization programs today.

Then, in 1981, the Carters were out of office. I was still working with the Centers for Disease Control as much as I could, and so was Rosalynn even though the Carters were back in Georgia after being defeated for a second term. We still did some national-level work with the Centers for Disease Control because Dr. Foege stayed on for two years under President Ronald Reagan. Reagan wanted him to stay longer, but he went to the Carter Center to work on children's health affairs. Dr. Foege was their executive director for years. And through that, we have continued our work.

By 1982, we had gotten the laws changed so that all children entering school had to be fully immunized. But there were still pockets, many pockets, where children weren't getting their needed vaccines. To get something like that done—to have it be effective, to have it work and be accountable—is so cumbersome. It takes so much work and so much time to get accomplished. I was still working in that area, but in 1982, I started full-time with Peace Links. I really was concentrating on that until one day in early 1990 when Rosalynn called me. We had had that big epidemic of measles that killed nearly 120 people, many of whom were infants, between 1989 and 1990. We realized that while we had done a wonderful thing by encouraging the passage of school laws requiring immunizations by kindergarten entry, we had perhaps shifted people's opinions or their thinking away from the early immunizations needed by age two.

In fact, children should receive the majority of their shots by their second birthday, but our work had encouraged the perception that it was all right to wait until school age. So this big population of kids from birth to five years of age was left vulnerable to measles, and in that epidemic many of them got struck down and died. That's when Rosalynn called and said, "Betty, what are we going to do about all these babies dying?"

We had talked about our role after that measles epidemic, and we accepted the fact that we had helped create the situation with our school-age immunization work. I asked, "How much time can you give me?" And she said, "Whatever it takes, but I am leaving for China tomorrow." She tells this as another story at our dog-and-pony shows. She says, "When I came back, Betty already had an office, a director, and oh, I don't know what all."

We were set up. Dr. Foege was at the Carter Center working on children's health issues, and he had guided and helped me. We had already established a name for the program: Every Child By Two (ECBT). Rosalynn and I visited every state over the next two years, trying to get the health departments, the schools, and the day cares to look into the issue. We wanted to get laws in place to make sure children in every day care, even in homes, were immunized. We wanted to shift people's thinking, so we held workshops and invited people through each state's governor's office. We would have two or three workshops in a state and go visit the lot of them.

This was all being guided by Dr. Foege, who understood organizing the way Nell Balkman did; she was still the honcho of how to organize. They adopted my Arkansas program as a model for national immunization, and ECBT followed right along. I guess you would say I have been instrumental in shaping the way we immunize kids. I pushed Rosalynn to be president of ECBT, and she has always shown up whenever I needed her. And as I have said many times, what else do you need besides a former First Lady and somebody with tenacity? I think our most important contribution was the encouragement of the development of immunization coalitions in communities throughout the nation. This model has been instrumental in ensuring that local-level needs are met through the involvement of committed individuals who can assess the needs and steer the resources toward achieving their goals. We remain involved in supporting coalitions at the local level to this day.

ECBT has evolved tremendously over the past twenty years. We have continued to remain active in establishing and supporting federal and state legislation to enhance vaccine delivery. We have developed dozens of educational programs for health care providers, coalitions, and the public. We developed the first immunization-focused newsletter back in 1996 when the Internet was just coming into use and subsequently one of the first immunization-focused websites (www.ecbt.org), which is still in existence today. For the past ten years ECBT has played a leading role in educating the media and the public about the continued safety of vaccines in the face of false allegations that they cause illnesses such as multiple sclerosis, autism, and other disorders. ECBT's newest website and social media campaign (www.vaccinateyourbaby.org) has been credited by media, journalists, and newspapers nationwide as a credible source for vaccine safety information for families seeking to wade through the abundance of misinformation available on the Web. Rosalynn and I have been all over the country trying to counter this autism myth, and I still do a lot of work on that. Our organization has always remained lean (we typically maintain three staff people, including Amy Pisani, who is very sharp and dedicated and has been the executive director since 1998). In fact, our partners often marvel at the impact we continue to have on policy, public education, and so forth.

One issue we have been working on since the late 1970s was getting state laws in place to govern immunization for day cares. Without rules or regulations, one infant could come in with measles or any other disease and expose the whole day care. Now in many states, children have to be fully immunized before they can get into day care or Head Start programs because we got those laws in place. You learn so much about states and how they work, and you just wish sometimes that everything would be under federal control. But that would have drawbacks, too. I think we should have public health clinics in the schools, but even Rosalynn didn't support this. I believe that since the children are already in school, they could get health care there, but not many people supported the idea. There are school clinics now successfully running in many places throughout the country; however, with our focus on the young child, we have learned that it is not the best venue for universal vaccination. However, teens who are in need of booster shots and shots to prevent human papillomavirus and meningitis are often able to attain these vaccines through such clinics. You just learn so much through years of experience.

Another issue we worked on at the same time that still needs attention was getting money to the states to develop computerized immunization information systems. A lot of states got money to buy computers, but there was no mandate to use them for immunization records. Another similar issue was getting states to help private doctors computerize their records. Some states are just now starting to do that, and so much more is needed.

I think states, especially the state legislatures, have an extremely important role in immunization. After all, they are looked to as legalists, they make laws, and they are charged with looking after people, their constituents. They need to keep themselves informed of all the safety issues, the exemption requirements, and the state's investment into the immunization strategies. Legislators need to stay informed about the addition of new vaccines and help formulate laws so that those vaccines are given before school entry (including college entry) and also for other day care situations. Legislators play an extremely important role, and so I think that it would be in their interest to stay well informed. There are many places, including ECBT, that they can get the information.

Now things are better and people understand more, but when we started, in a city like Houston, only 14 percent of children from birth to two years of age were immunized. In some places nationally, rates were even lower, and no state had a very high level. Most young children weren't immunized; parents waited until they were six and then went to preschool or school clinics to start the immunization records. Now, with the laws in place, that percentage ranges in the nineties for immunization by age two.

Rosalynn and I have been a good working team, which is why I have stayed on it, stayed in it, and stayed committed. With her presence, we can get an audience with any governor or state legislature. Many people know me through my husband's being a governor and senator. I am not saying that people know me because really they have known Dale. He has been out there fighting for them to get vaccines in their states. That has been a really good working team, too—his work and then my tenacity!

CONNECTIONS

EVERY CHILD BY TWO, BETTY BUMPERS, AND CHILDREN'S HEALTH POLICY

AMY PISANI, EXECUTIVE DIRECTOR, EVERY CHILD BY TWO

Organizational History

Since the founding of Every Child By Two (ECBT) nearly twenty years ago, our staff and cofounders have traveled to every state in the nation (most more than once) to highlight the critical importance of vaccines. ECBT's cofounders, former First Lady Rosalynn Carter and former First Lady of Arkansas Betty Bumpers, are dedicated to reducing child morbidity and mortality through timely immunization. Inspired by the dedication of these two ladies, ECBT's staff and board of directors strive to develop and facilitate programs to ensure that every child in our nation receive their primary immunizations by the age of two.

Today's public health infrastructure consists of a combination of federal, state, local, nonprofit, and private entities that strive to maintain high immunization rates and universal access to vaccine for children, adolescents, and adults. However, in the 1970s, our nation had not yet galvanized efforts to defeat vaccine-preventable diseases. At that time, the Centers for Disease Control (CDC) approached Betty Bumpers, who had begun her tenure as First Lady of Arkansas, to request that she assist in raising her state's immunization rates, which were below 45 percent. Mrs. Bumpers responded within weeks by galvanizing every resource in Arkansas—state agencies, religious organizations, agricultural extension workers, and many other groups—thereby establishing one of the first immunization coalitions in the country. Immunization rates soared, and her accomplishments were heralded by CDC director Dr. William Foege who requested that she encourage other states to create similar programs. She responded to the CDC's request by presenting her program at governors' conferences and many other gubernatorial venues. Along with several other First Ladies, Rosalynn Carter, First Lady of Georgia, took on the cause in her home state.

When Jimmy Carter was elected president, Mrs. Bumpers, who had come to Washington several years prior when her husband was elected to the U.S. Senate, contacted the new administration to explain the deficiencies in the U.S. immunization program and to request that immunizations become a priority of the Carter administration. As a result, in 1977, a national childhood immunization initiative was announced with two goals: (1) attainment of childhood immunization levels of 90 percent by October 1979 and (2) establishment of a permanent system to provide comprehensive immunization services to the 3 million children born in the United States each year. Dr. Joseph Califano, secretary of health, education, and welfare (the U.S. Department of Health, Education, and Welfare is now called the U.S. Department of Health and Human Services), outlined a program requiring increased federal support for immunizations, increased involvement of volunteers, increased public awareness and education activities, and increased cooperation between government agencies.[12]

At the same time, Rosalynn Carter and Betty Bumpers began the successful campaign to encourage school-entry laws among the states. They have since been credited with efforts to enact laws in every state mandating vaccination verification prior to school entry. As a result, the United States currently boasts an immunization rate of more than 90 percent for children entering school. Once this was accomplished, they (and many others) believed that they had vaccine-preventable diseases under control. However, the measles outbreaks of 1989–1991, which claimed the lives of 123 and resulted in 55,000 reported cases, many of whom were unvaccinated preschoolers, proved them wrong. In response to this epidemic, Carter and Bumpers joined together to form ECBT to reeducate the public about the need to complete the major series of vaccines by the age of two, when children are at greatest risk of contracting many of the diseases. The official mission of ECBT is "to increase awareness of the need for timely immunization and develop a systematic method of locating and vaccinating all children into the future."

ECBT's initial strategy was to travel to every state in the country to encourage the development of immunization coalitions, garner commitments from high-level stakeholders, and alert the public about the consequences of low immunization rates and effects of vaccine-preventable diseases. The trips were an enormous success. In state after state, publicity of the purpose of the visits by local news stations and print journals far exceeded expectations. However, it rapidly became clear that efforts required action by more than just public health employees. Raising the awareness of the public, particularly among young parents who had not experienced the devastating effects of many of the diseases, and ensuring access to and availability of immunization services would require a joint effort by those in power to make the necessary changes. In many of these states, the first formal immunization coalitions were developed, many of which continue to thrive today.

As Bill Clinton came into office in 1993, Dale and Betty Bumpers, who had maintained their roots in Arkansas, were instrumental in encouraging the Clinton administration to develop the Childhood Immunization Initiative. According to Dr. Walter Orenstein, former director of the CDC's National Immunization Program, "This infusion of funds and commitment by national leaders helped the nation achieve 90 percent immunization coverage of preschool children."

At the state level, ECBT has a long history of working with legislators beginning during the Carter administration and in a concerted manner since the inception of ECBT in 1991. State visits by Carter and Bumpers regularly include interaction with key members of state legislatures and other stakeholders to discuss the particular challenges of each state. ECBT has also presented at numerous events sponsored by the National Conference of State Legislatures, which is a bipartisan organization serving the legislators and staffs of the nation's fifty states, commonwealths, and territories. ECBT staff, cofounders, and board members have presented on the issues of state versus federal budgeting for immunization activities, immunization information system support, vaccine safety, enforcement of vaccine requirements for schools, and the overall value of vaccines. In addition, ECBT's cofounders have addressed members of the National Governors Association during several annual meetings.

In 2008, ECBT initiated the largest campaign in the history of our organization: Vaccinate Your Baby. This multifaceted public health education campaign targets the entire U.S. population with messages about vaccine safety and the importance of vaccinating children in accordance with the recommended immunization schedule of the Advisory Committee on Immunization Practices. The campaign directly addresses misinformation about the safety of vaccines and directs the public to credible research and science-based immunization information, housed on the Vaccinate Your Baby campaign website, to ensure that they are making proper health care decisions for themselves and their families.

The Vaccinate Your Baby campaign has generated significant coverage in magazines and online mentions/blogs, such as *People*, *Cookie*, *Parenting*, *CBS* and *ABC News Online*, *NBC News*, the *New York Post*, the *New York Times*, the *New York Daily News*, the *Seattle Times*, the *Chicago Tribune*, the *Los Angeles Times*, the *Washington Post*, the *Washington Times*, and *USA Today*. ECBT serves as a reliable/expeditious source of information for an increasing number of print and television reporters. Producers and reporters from *NBC News*, *ABC Evening News*, *ABC's Good Morning America*, and *USA Today* are in contact with ECBT staff on regular basis to ensure fact-based immunization reporting.

ECBT also produced two new public service announcements, featuring Amanda Peet, that express the message that the public should trust in their doctors for vaccine advice. The Vaccinate Your Baby campaign has reached more than 153 million people via print and online stories, 10 million television program/news viewers, and 500 million PSA viewers of the previously mentioned public service announcements.

Because of these efforts and others, the U.S. immunization rates are the highest achieved in the nation's history,[13] resulting in record-low morbidity and mortality from vaccine-preventable diseases.[14] Betty Bumpers was instrumental in immunization networks and, along with cofounder Rosalynn Carter, the establishment of ECBT. Their work for the health of children and adults has saved lives and promoted well-being.

NOTES

1. Betty Bumpers, "Article for *Unitarian Universalist World*," manuscript, July 7, 1986, Peace Links Records Addendum (MC 907a), series 1, subseries 4, box 7, folder 7-9, Special Collections, University of Arkansas Libraries, Fayetteville, 2.
2. Materials within quotation marks are from Bumpers's speeches or writings, cited as endnotes below. Materials outside quotation marks are derived from interviews with Betty Bumpers by Anna and Jennie Eblen, August 29–31, 2005; May 14, 2006; October 2–6, 2007; and February 24–26, 2009.
3. Betty Bumpers, "Memorable Days," speech manuscript (n.d.); Betty Bumpers Childhood Immunization Project Papers (MC 1204), box 5, folder 2, Special Collections, University of Arkansas Libraries, Fayetteville, 1–2.
4. Betty Bumpers, "Remarks," acceptance speech, 2005 Induction, National Women's Hall of Fame, Seneca Falls, New York, October 8, 2005; Peace Links Records Addendum (unprocessed), Special Collections, University of Arkansas Libraries, Fayetteville.
5. Bumpers, paraphrased from "Memorable Days," 1.
6. Bumpers, "Remarks," 1.
7. Bumpers, "Memorable Days," 2.
8. "Voluntary Action Center," www.handsonnetwork.org/files/resources/VCs_A_History_of_America.pdf (accessed November 13, 2010).
9. "Voluntary Action Center," www.handsonnetwork.org/files/resources/VCs_A_History_of_America.pdf (accessed November 13, 2010); National Volunteer Action Center, renamed Voluntary Action Center.
10. President Richard Nixon's secretary of health, education, and welfare; secretary of defense; and attorney general.
11. MD in pediatrics and surgeon general under President Bill Clinton.
12. Stanley A. Plotkin and Walter A. Orenstein, *Vaccines*, 3rd ed. (Philadelphia: W. B. Saunders, 1999).
13. Centers for Disease Control and Prevention, "National Immunization Survey 2008 Table Data," www.cdc.gov/vaccines/stats-surv/nis/data/tables_2008.htm (accessed July 2010.
14. Sandra Roush and Trudy Murphy, "Historical Comparisons of Morbidity and Mortality for Vaccine-Preventable Diseases in the United States," *Journal of the American Medical Association* 298, no. 18 (2007): 2155–63.

THREE

Linking for Peace

> And we also felt that by using our voices, as credible, highly visible women on this issue, it would encourage others to find their own voices and be heard.[1]

CONVERSATIONS WITH BETTY[2]

"My entry into the peace movement came late. . . . Starting a large new project was the last thing I had expected to be doing at age 57. Although I now applaud those visionaries who were a part of the peace movement in the Sixties, I was not one of them. I was then a housewife in Charleston, Arkansas (population 1,700), driving three children to their activities and lessons, teaching art part-time and being a volunteer for everything."[3] "The lessons which I learned about grassroots organizing . . . were to serve me well when I started Peace Links."[4]

"I founded Peace Links Worldwide out of the belief that the special gifts of women were needed as never before in leadership roles throughout our society. I still believe that. But I came to recognize an even deeper need. It's not enough for us to bring forth the best women leaders and the best men leaders. Somehow, someway we need to find a way to link the positive feminine and masculine characteristics of leadership into an integrated whole. That means that we have to share the best of ourselves with each other."[5]

"The idea that I should be doing something to prevent nuclear war grew out of a conversation I had with my daughter, Brooke, then a college student, when we were on our way back to Washington in 1981. We had just crossed the Clinch River in eastern Tennessee, when Brooke confronted me with the question of how our family would get back together if a nuclear disaster occurred. . . . The threat of nuclear war was an all-pervasive theme, enveloping everything that was happening in Washington. Nobody really talked about it the way Brooke had, but the arms buildup was decidedly underway."[6]

"I came to the peace movement out of despair, but I stayed out of hope. A bishop in Iowa whom I met when I first started Peace Links said to me: 'This country has had three great decisions to make during its history. The first was to decide whether it would remain a colony or become a free nation. The second was whether we would tolerate slavery or would all be free. The third is now whether we will become extinct or learn to live peaceably together.' [It seemed to me that] we had an opportunity, and that what each of us did in that moment and for the rest of our lives could determine the course of the future. We owed it to our children, our community, our country, our planet to make sure that our voices were heard and sustained."[7]

When I started Peace Links, I just dared to bring up nuclear war and be outraged at what was happening. I was privileged to be living in Washington, where I could go to seminars and where women were involved in groups like Women's International League for Peace and Freedom. I went to brown-bag lunches and heard some of the more sophisticated people, like Nancy Ramsey, who consulted in Washington, D.C., about national security and was the first director for the Americans for SALT [Strategic Arms Limitation Treaty, or SALT II]. I was also learning some information from hearing my husband talk about what was going on.

I knew that Dale got off the Senate Armed Services Committee because, as he said, "You know I just can't deal with some of that conversation they're having about developing a bomb that would kill people more than it would destroy buildings." This was back before some of the bombs we have now existed. He said, "I just can't take that kind of thing, and I'm going to get off that committee."

I dared to start talking about the issue because my daughter and other young people were so attuned to it. I was flying back and forth to Arkansas pretty often, and I'd talk to everybody on the airplane. People would look at me, like, "Well, have you fallen out of a high tree or something?" It was unusual, especially for women, to question what men were doing to us with this war business—all of these weapons.

Peace Links started in Arkansas when I was talking to a lot of friends about my ideas. I said a lot of times in conversation that I had just assumed that the men who knew about war and weapons and such things were taking care of us. Then I took a look at it, and I thought, "This ain't the way I want to be taken care of." Other women were like me—it was just that I came to the awareness suddenly because of my daughter's remarks. That was the reason I got started, and it became an awakening to women. I'd go to any group, to small women's clubs, all over the state, all over the country, and it was a revelation to them.

In my experience, very few men can shift their thinking—do out-of-the-box thinking—but women are very capable of that. It's as though there's some mechanism in men's heads, and even though they get the information, they just don't hear it, but women do. An analogy I've used many times is, how many men do you know who can hip a baby, stir a sauce, settle an argument in the living room between older siblings, and plan next week's club meeting all at one time? Women got it when I said, "I thought men were taking care of us." I would say this in a way that got to the heart of the problem, like my dad used to talk.

After a summer in Arkansas, I decided I wanted to do something similar to what I had done with immunizations for children. Before, while I was trying to get the Arkansas immunization model as a national model, I had met a young friend who helped me get in contact with the governors' wives. This young woman had been in the Peace Corps, and when I told her about this peace idea, she said, "I know the first person you need to talk to." She meant Debbie Harding, who was with Peace Links from the beginning. So back in Washington, I invited Debbie to lunch, and she brought along this young man, Rob. I talked about my ideas, and they helped me get into funding. She and Rob had gone with Rosalynn Carter to Biafra, so they were well connected in the networks here in Washington. Debbie had stayed in touch with lots of the Peace Corps volunteers, and she was trying to put back together the Peace Corps list because the list of original Peace Corps volunteers had been destroyed. She was working out of Sargent Shriver's law office during Watergate, and that later became our first Peace Links office.

Debbie was on the Peace Links board forever (chair of the board), and she was tough on us. She made sure that we were careful with money and fund-raising. She was pretty good on programs committee in terms of ideas. Debbie and Rob suggested the first executive director, Nancy Graham, who had been Debbie's Peace Corps director. Nancy went with me to start helping organize in Arkansas, but I realized she really didn't have the same idea I did. Hers was a more sophisticated concept than I wanted, and I decided that Nancy just wasn't the right executive director.

When I got back to Washington, D.C., I had a reception, and a whole bunch of other congressional wives came to it. I think the fact that I spoke up started things, and it helped when I found Carol Williams, who volunteered with Peace Links for a long time. Carol told me Laurie Daschle would be ideal for the director's position. Laurie was divorcing [Senator Tom Daschle], and the Peace Links job seemed right for her. The women I talked to all had stories about their kids. For instance, Teresa Heinz [Kerry] told me that my story about Brooke motivated her to get involved. She was a congressional wife, and she called and said, "Betty, I have a Brooke story to tell you." She had heard I was going to sponsor a gathering, and she described how her three boys were playing out in the backyard of their home in Georgetown. "As all moms do, I was listening to their conversation, and they were digging a hole thinking they were going to China. But their conversation turned to, "How deep a hole do you think we'd have to dig for us to crawl in and be safe from a nuclear bomb?" She saw the same thing I did and asked to hold the luncheon at her house and cosponsor it with me. That's how I got the response that I did, and most of the congressional wives came to the lunch. Everybody had a similar story: that their children brought them to it. By saying, "This is not the way I want to be taken care of," I brought out how they were feeling.

Carol [spouse of Montana congressman Pat Williams] had started volunteering right away. And finally we put her on the payroll [executive director] when we had enough money because she worked at it so long as a volunteer. I think she got 172 congressional spouses to lend their name to our Peace Links initiative. That was a very valuable tool. It was a big gift to us for the spouses to give us their names. For people in a state, seeing that their congressional representatives or spouses were on that list gave us a lot of credibility, and that's what Carol did by recruiting congressional wives.

Dale was very busy and going back to Arkansas frequently. Brooke went away to college. I had the empty-nest feeling, so I took off. Dale didn't mind if I was gone, and I'd try to schedule my trips conveniently for him. I was home an adequate amount, but he was so busy, and he didn't know how to relax like I did. He grew up with that old Christian ethic to just work as hard as you can at whatever job you're doing.

Everybody knew this was the first time that a Senate wife had ever reared her head up to do something so controversial. Randy Forsberg's nuclear freeze idea traveled like wildfire among the people in Washington and nationally. There were several other peace organizations all popping up about the same time, like WAND [Women's Action for Nuclear Disarmament, later Women's Action for New Directions], so I was on their advisory committee, and we would cooperate with them. I didn't try to compete or try to take over anything of theirs. A lot of peace groups were very challenging, very possessive of their organizations. They didn't want to be cooperative. But I had no pride in that way. I just wanted all of us to work together.

As I learned more about nuclear weapons I got so upset. Being raised by a father who convinced us that we could do anything we wanted to do in this world if we worked hard enough, I worked at it. You've got to work hard. The fact that I dared just to talk about these things was unusual, and my husband got pretty upset a few times. You can imagine a senator's wife talking about peace like this. At one big fund-raiser for one of his Senate races, somebody yelled from the back of the crowd, "Senator, ain't your wife's involvement with that peace outfit and all gonna hurt your chances for reelection?" Dale, thank God, said something like, "Only among those who favor whooping cough or nuclear war." The crowd laughed, and that served notice to every newspaper, every editorial board in the country. You would get laughed out of town with that kind of attack, so they weren't going to go anyplace with it. He knew it was going to come up, but he is very clever that way, fast on the repartee.

"I spent . . . years of my life criss-crossing this country from one end to the other, and circling the globe as well, trying to find some answers to the hard, hard problems that confronted our whole human family. I did not do this because I am a natural born crusader. I am not. This role was very hard for me. I did it because I'm a mother, and because I had a child who awakened me to the peril that we were all facing through her own fears and anxieties.

"Dr. Robert J. Lifton, professor of psychiatry at Yale University, says: 'The imagery of nuclear extinction begins in young people at the age of four or five—it doesn't wait for adulthood—they can't help but take in this imagery.' Children everywhere were sounding their fearful cry to the person they most depended upon for nurturing and care—Mother. Awakened by the cries of their children, women all over the earth rose up out of some kind of deep, instinctive need to protect their children on a vast, planetary scale. I've sat and talked with such women from Florida and Montana, Pennsylvania and California, Arkansas and Kansas—mothers from England, Germany, and the Soviet Union—all of us linked together by a common bond of maternal love and the desire for the common good of our children."[8]

"Peace is not exclusively a women's issue. Many good men were involved from the beginning. But the leadership which emerged among women on this issue, I believe, was a major force in bringing a mind-shift—a shift in our thinking—which moved us away from world war and toward promising alternatives.

"Women have historically played a role in bringing change to our society usually without fanfare or recognition. What women have done in the peace movement in the past may never make it into the history books, but I am confident that our leadership helped change history. Women approach the struggle for peace with a passion and determination which make it impossible for their voices to be ignored. We make no apologies for the fact that we had a different perspective from that of many men on how the world's problems should be addressed. We acknowledge the fact that we tend to think relationally and to see the world as interconnected. It was easy to find our voices when we were talking about the families of the world that we cared about.

"We knew that we had to speak out to stop the rapid escalation toward nuclear war because our sixth sense told us that our children—and our homes on this planet—were in jeopardy. We knew that no other issue mattered unless alternatives to nuclear war were found. We knew our children would have no futures unless alternatives to nuclear war were found. And when our children were at risk, it was hard to keep us silent.

We found our voices with peace ribbons, with banners, with quilts, with demonstrations, with poems, with songs, with telling our own stories. We brought to our efforts in the peace movement the persistence, the capacity for repetitive work, the tenacity, the emotions and questions which it took to make a leap of consciousness. Women's voices were not only heard, but were sustained because our daughters and sons and grandchildren joined in."[9]

"These women in towns and cities across the country learned just how much difference their efforts made on the important issue of nuclear war. What they built for themselves and others . . . was influence and therefore, hope. We knew there were alternatives to mutually assured destruction. We also knew that together we could find them.

"Each year we had seen more and more of our wealth being used for weaponry we knew we could never use and survive. And each year we saw less attention being paid to the education and health care of our children. We realized that our national security for the future lay not in building exotic weapon systems but in the care and education we gave our children. And the number of people who wanted to see those priorities reordered grew . . . the women in Peace Links were part of that growing number and the dedication and ingenuity which they brought to their efforts for peace was impressive. They did not pretend to be experts in defense or arms issues but, as women, they did know a great deal about nurturing new life, about sharing power and about linking up with each other on important issues."[10]

In the meantime, there was a big brouhaha, and I got called a communist [by Senator Denton on the floor of the U.S. Senate]. That put us on the map here in Washington. I don't know exactly how we got all the connections with different groups all over the country. There was an article in the *Parade* magazine, and that's probably how some groups reached us. There were the contacts that I had with the governor's wives. We worked through Laurie and the connections of congressional wives, and then I traveled and recruited women. We would go out to communities and speak. You don't have to be an expert; all you have to do is break through that language that they shut us out with. [We would] look it up in a little handbook that was put out to demystify that language, like what's an ICBM [intercontinental ballistic missile]? Sometimes we had military officers who would come to debate us. The military people tried to use technical vocabulary that would shut us out because it was a vocabulary we didn't know and didn't relate to. Once you set up the problem in a new way, you rip the veil away. It's like the story of the emperor who had no clothes. Women are capable of reconsidering; they'll say, "Yes, well, I never thought about it that way." When enough women shift their thinking because they are the ones who protect and guide, who take care of their families, things will change things. As my husband has said, "You just turn it over to a woman. When it comes to their families and defending their children, they'll attack a circle saw."

One of the last questions I always asked, when a general was up there debating with this long spiel of how special these weapons were, was, "Yes, but where are you taking us? We understand all that you said, but where is that taking us? What good are these weapons that we never use and we are building them up?" They never, ever got it. I'll tell you men can't shift their thinking. The generals just build more and more. It doesn't matter whether we use the weapons or not. Men are on that track, and that's where we're going.

The Peace Panel concept was a panel of women who got up and talked about how they felt about an issue. With four or five other women sitting up there with them, they could give that little speech. The idea came out of the crisis in Little Rock, Arkansas, over school segregation, when we were trying to get the schools reopened all around the state. The original panels, called "A Panel of American Women," would pick a woman from about every ethnic group who'd go to the schools, the clubs, and organizations. Panelists would stand up and talk about how they felt about discrimination. This was fifty years ago, and Jews were still discriminated against, so Jewish women and black women would talk about how discrimination made them feel and what a problem it was. These were highly credible women.

Later in Peace Links, Elinor Bedell, another congressional wife, told her story many times. She was very shy, and she said, "I hid behind my mother's skirts growing up. Then I married Burke and hid behind his pant legs until I met Betty Bumpers." Elinor's daughter and son-in-law had two young boys, and the couple decided to take off, carrying the boys in backpacks, and see the world before some nuclear holocaust destroyed it. That kind of shook Elinor up, and she came to the Peace Links meeting. Women at the meetings knew I was not a trained, eloquent speaker. I was just an ordinary mom, and I kept saying, "People just need to meet someone who will speak up. You can't sit at home in a nice house; you need to get up and do something about it. I don't care what it is, just do something." I later took that panel idea and turned it into this empowerment workshop. I look back now and wonder how I had the guts. I would just go into a group of people and I would ask them, "How do you feel about the fact that we have such a huge number of nuclear weapons?" I'd just pick somebody out. They'd articulate something. I'd ask six or eight of them, with Carol or somebody up onstage, writing their points down. I'd ask several other questions, and out of the seven or so answers to the questions, Carol would pick five women. I would call them up to the front. I'd say, "You come up here and turn that answer into a speech." They'd say, "*Me*? Oh." But then they were thrilled to death, it was flattering. And they would come up.

It empowered them for us to verify that they had said something important, and they had. People like Carol would pick up the ones with a nugget of a good speech. We'd give them a few minutes to prepare, and it was outstanding how they could take that little nugget and turn it into a speech. Sometimes I would get into hot water, but somehow I'd get out.

We supported each other in those Peace Panels when we presented at women's clubs or meetings of women's organizations. One of our best illustrations was about the outrageous number of weapons, and it started with a single BB dropped into a metal dish. In that demonstration, Elinor learned how to talk about nuclear war when she slowly poured BBs into a metal dish to illustrate the number of nuclear weapons. I'll bet she did that demonstration a thousand times, and it helped her to overcome her shyness. We held training courses and peace rallies that helped a lot of women. I loved that kind of thing; I just loved doing all that.

What I strove to do was visit local Peace Links to talk about what was happening on the national scene: the buildup of more and more nuclear weapons that we didn't need. It was in the paper every day about how many it would take to blow us all apart. Local Peace Links worried, "How can you say that when military leaders say we need this?" And I said, "Because it is just stupidity. Men simply are not relating to it."

You could see that most of the women connected. I said, "I can't come here and organize this and tell you what to do and how, but you can start. I am trying to empower you to take this into your own hands, organize, and do it the way you want to do it. What we want is a Peace Day. And you need to put Peace Day on the agenda of your groups." If they said, "The agenda is full," I would say, "Ask for an add-on. Take on this issue if you want to stand up in the face of what is happening to you. Your money is being spent on nuclear weapons, and it is not making you safer. It's making you more unsafe."

I did this in every community, and then I would just walk away and leave it to them. And I would say, "I can't tell you how to do it because you live here." It empowered women to think, "Yeah, I know how and I can." And they did. All I did was try to come back in, praise them for what a great job they had done, and offer whatever national assistance we could. What resources I could gather for the national office—the money I got—I tried to share with the local Peace Links. At the beginning, I *was* the national office of Peace Links. We very seldom had money. But we would support the local groups in other ways—in materials, in ideas, in cooperation.

"We did not tell them what to do [in local Peace Links.] We simply presented the issues and trusted them to come up with their own ways on dealing with them locally. They exceeded all our expectations, from turning out whole cities for the 1980s Soviet women's visits to registering voters in numbers large enough to change election outcomes."[11]

"Peace Links brought . . . women from the Soviet Union to this country to visit with American women in an effort to promote understanding. The discussions were often open and frank, especially when they involved the ways women were treated at home and in the workplace. Differences over our political systems occasionally surfaced but we found that, as women, we had far more in common than we had in things that separated us."[12]

We also had our Pen Pal project with correspondence between Americans and Russian pen pals. It was so successful and brought a lot of attention. Many, many wonderful stories came out of that. I sent about 10,000 letters that we could not get translated to the University of Arkansas Peace Links archives. One of the heart-wrenching things was a lot of letters about Chernobyl from people in Ukraine and downwind. You'd hear problems, within a few years, with children who were starving; they were innocent victims. There was medical help that we were able to get to some of the people.

We started conflict resolution and empowerment workshops, like Listen Up, for high school students, and some of them are still going. For Listen Up, we interviewed kids to find out what made them feel safer. It wasn't metal detectors or police. They were ticked because metal detectors made them have to walk around the school building and in one side. They did not like having police on the grounds, but they wanted to learn how to be safe with each other. Some of these conflict management workshops are still going today. I heard that a lot of organizations had taken those empowerment activities and models and expanded them into really sophisticated things. If I had been smarter, if we had all been a little smarter and more sophisticated and had the money, who knows? We could have done a lot of things because we had some fabulous ideas just out of groups around my kitchen table early on. We called it the Kitchen Cabinet. We were just coming up with ideas; we'd talk, roll ideas around, try them out, and then we'd finally come up with a plan from a group effort. But we did spend so much time trying to raise money.

Within a few years, our early executive director, Laurie Daschle, had to leave because she had to equip herself to educate her children, so she went to law school. And then we went through a series of executive directors before Carol came along and stabilized it, but money was just always a problem. We had the holiday gala to raise funds and gave the Eleanor Roosevelt Living World Award to women leaders who contributed to peace and the survival of the planet: Hillary Clinton, Madeleine Albright, Rosalynn Carter, Coretta Scott King, Loret Ruppe, the ambassador to Norway who had directed the Peace Corps. We honored Valentina Tereshkova, the first cosmonaut, and the first award went to Gro Harlem Brundtland, prime minister of Norway. People loved having this kind of event at the holidays. I wanted our effort to be bipartisan, so I invited both Republicans and Democrats, and I was heartened by how readily they responded.

"In the late years of the twentieth century, we lived in a nuclear age, confronted by dangers never before known by humanity. We needed all the strengths of the whole human race working together. The problems we faced were not male or female, black or white, Christian or Jew, American or Russian. They were human problems. They involved us all, and they threatened us all. We worked together. We tried to listen and learn from each other.

"Why was this so hard? It was the listening and learning that seemed hardest of all. I was continuously amazed at how the very word 'peace' threatened so many people. They were terrified by it. With ears plugged and minds closed, they lashed out with angry words and bitter denunciations. I've probably been called every name in the book, all the way from the floor of Congress to half the truck stops in Arkansas and Mississippi. At best I was labeled naive, and at worst I was called a communist and a traitor. To those who questioned my loyalty to this country, I sincerely questioned their faith in the very democracy they so loudly claimed to defend."[13]

"We showed that the democratic system works best when more people participate in it. What you and I think and say does make a difference to leaders in determining the priorities of this country. Peace Links helped show that movement toward peace was possible if enough of us believed in it and insisted that our leaders spend as much time, effort and money to bring it about as they spent on preparing for future wars."[14]

"When the atom was first split in the nineteen forties, Albert Einstein said it changed everything save man's thinking. The time came when we had no choice but to move toward that major mind-shift. Every mother knows there are better ways than fighting to resolve conflicts. We insisted that our leaders also find those better ways."[15]

"This did not mean that we jumped into instant Utopia. And it certainly did not mean that we immediately threw away all our weapons and place ourselves at the mercy of [aggressors]. It just meant that we recognized that the path we were upon was fraught with danger and that we began to look for another way. Maybe we will never reach the point where we can live without nuclear weapons. I don't know. I only know that the situation we were in during the Cold War was the equivalent of two boys standing waist deep in a tub of gasoline holding lighted matches arguing. We had to blow out the matches. We had to begin somewhere. And the only place that I knew to begin was with the idea of hope. We believed that there was another way. We believed that there were answers to the problems we seek. We believed we had role in the future.

"We trusted ourselves to grow beyond the old ways of war and aggression for solving problems. We trusted our nation would lead us in a true democratic spirit and would not be afraid to listen to the diverse voices in search of those ways. We listened to each other and were not afraid because I thought one way and you thought another. If we can ever learn to really stop and listen, I'm betting that we can discover that our ways are not as far apart as we had thought. We can listen and then feel ourselves joined in a bond of common fears, dreads, dreams and hopes.

"And when we reach this point, I have a feeling that we will at last discover the real secret of peace. [We discovered in Peace Links that] peace is not a far off thing dependent upon the whims of Moscow and Washington. We found that peace is a very intimate, personal thing, dependent upon the will of you and me. Together we made a difference."[16]

CONNECTIONS

EXCERPTS FROM "AN OUNCE OF DISSENSION," *ARKANSAS TIMES*, AUGUST 1985

MARA LEVERITT, SENIOR EDITOR, *ARKANSAS TIMES*, AUTHOR OF *DEVIL'S KNOT*

Betty Bumpers spent her term as First Lady of Arkansas looking after the state's children. While her husband and elected officials wrestled with big-ticket matters of state, she was in the background saying to parents, in effect, "Now have you made sure the children have taken their medicine?" . . .

Now that she's in Washington as wife of Arkansas's senior United States senator, Bumpers feels the same ire as she watches the nations of the world amass their stockpiles of nuclear weapons. She'd still rather see the effort put into prevention, and characteristically, she's doing something about it. . . .

Betty Bumpers has grayed a little since she was the First Lady. Now that she's past sixty, she says she's given up trying to be glamorous and strives mainly for clean. It's not true—one never gives up—but the remark, imparted as a kind of sisterly aside, is typical of her; it's the kind of disarming self-ribbing a woman of airs cannot manage.

Bumpers is speaking this afternoon to the Arkansas Young Democrats in the dining room of the Little Rock Hilton. She's back home and enjoying it, but her message is the same one she has carried all over the country. In the past three years, Betty Bumpers has traveled like a campaigner, organizing supporters and speaking to almost anyone who will listen—first to a few friends in Arkansas and Washington, then to women at neighborhood coffees, then to religious assemblies, men's civic-club luncheons, teenagers, and congressmen. Her subject is intensely political, and it's certainly controversial, but Betty Bumpers is not going to all this effort to get anyone elected. Rather, she has taken on the task of trying to dis-elect, if you will, the idea of continued nuclear escalation. . . . As the YDs [Young Democrats] quietly spoon at their desserts, Bumpers begins with a clear and level voice her warning against the dangers of nuclear proliferation.

"Too many people—and I was one of them—think there's somebody out there taking care of the world for you." As straightforwardly as she talks of her age, she tells the group how for years she assumed somebody at the top had things under control, how she believed that elected leaders were somehow graced with the needed wisdom at their swearings-in, and how she voted for a good part of her life however her father and husband advised.

She acknowledges that it was not until her husband became governor that she realized the utterly human nature of leadership, and not till she moved with him to Washington that she understood the human frailty that's part of the fabric of even our own representative form of government. "God doesn't endow them with the power of knowing how to run the country," she says. Today she wonders at her own naivete at ever having thought otherwise. But she also realizes that she was not alone—that many women still believe "somebody" has things in hand, and that, just as she did, they've surrendered their own judgment to that belief. It's a startling and effective admission. In making it, she allies herself with many other American housewives and mothers. Her acknowledgment that she relied too much on a man touches every woman who has ever failed to credit her own good sense.

Betty Bumpers's "awakening," as she calls it, took place against the backdrop of Washington, amid debates on Capitol Hill and living-room discussions on international issues. She awoke to a world at risk—in greater jeopardy, she says, than she'd dared believe. She saw leaders, our own and others, exercising wisdom sometimes, groping with uncertainty at others, and sometimes being rash. As all this went on, the world's unprecedented capacity for destruction continued to grow. Ultimately, she awoke to the nightmare of mutually assured destruction and to the madness of the present alternative—a precarious peace under the shadow of nuclear war. Both courses, she concluded, were unacceptable. . . . Bumpers believes that survival is going to require . . . new methods of conflict resolution, new systems and institutions—and she sees it as her role these days to help bring that about. She uses military academies as an example. "They attract our brightest and best, and then they teach them how to wage war. What would happen if we developed just one academy that was devoted to training in the skills of peace?"

But she also warns that the demand for change won't come from Washington. It has started, she says, at the grassroots, with people who have concluded, as she has, that mankind is flirting with extinction. If that's revolutionary, she reminds her listeners, then so too at one time were the ideas of American independence, women's suffrage, and civil rights. . . .

The Young Democrats push back their chairs, rise, and applaud. She may have convinced none of them, or she may have inspired just one; she never can tell. All she knows is that in politics, as in nuclear physics, things happen once you reach a critical mass. Politically, that's the number of people who raise enough hell to get Congress to react. . . .

Peace Links is targeted at that broad swath called "middle America," and, more specifically, at middle-American women. . . . Peace Links is a response both to women's concerns and to their historical non-involvement in affairs of national security. "We don't want to exclude men in any way," she says. "But our goal is to persuade the leadership—and that is, after all, mostly men."

If the tableau of women trying to dispossess men of their warlike ways is a familiar one, the organization Bumpers has established to do that is not. There are no dues, no elected officers, and no regular meetings. Some members find the lack of a more formulated structure troublesome, but Bumpers considers Peace Links' loose, almost ad hoc arrangement not only appropriate but essential. . . . Instead of building an elaborate infrastructure of its own, Peace Links spreads by "linking" members in already-established organizations. . . .

Bumpers sees the issue of peace as an intellectual as well as an emotional one, and she looks for projects that will involve women at either or both levels. Nationally, members have instituted exchange tours between groups of American and Soviet women, participated in a "call-in" to the White House on President Reagan's birthday, and stitched a "peace quilt," under which they've invited every member of Congress to sleep for one night and then record their dreams of peace. (Thirty-seven senators already have. . . .)

Nationally, the biggest project by far has been one begun by a Denver housewife. It is the Peace Ribbon, a series of panels, each eighteen by thirty-six inches, on which women across the country have painted, embroidered, and appliqued symbols of peace and things they love. The ribbons have been used in several peaceful demonstrations throughout the United States, including one at the Arkansas State Capitol, and will eventually be combined and symbolically "wrapped" around the Pentagon. . . .

Peace Links has never advocated disarmament; only a de-escalation of the arms race. But even that stance has won it detractors. Three years ago, shortly after Bumpers had started the organization, Republican senator Jeremiah Denton of Alabama castigated it on the Senate floor. Denton, a former Navy admiral and pilot who spent seven years as a prisoner of war in North Vietnam, charged that Peace Links was guided by Communists. He was supported in that view by John East and Jesse Helms, senators from North Carolina.

Denton's charges were rebutted, and didn't damage Peace Links so much as publicize it. In a rare breach of protocol, several senators rose to condemn the accusation and speak in Betty Bumpers's defense. Among them were Democratic senator Gary Hart of Colorado—"I say to the senator from Alabama, 'Shame on you'"—and her husband, who noted for the record, "If people engage in appropriate activities to show their commitment to peace, if that becomes subversive, then we can kiss everything this country stands for goodbye. . . ."

In the end, all that Betty Bumpers and Peace Links are advocating is a similar mutuality in government. "I didn't know it," she says, "but I've been a feminist all my life. I'm not saying the world would be a better place if women had been running it all along, but I am saying it would be better if the decision-making had been shared, if they had taken us into their counsel—if we had put as much effort into trying to find ways *not* to kill as we put into finding ways to kill."

PEACE LINKS NORTH CAROLINA: BETTY'S INFLUENCES FROM A GRASSROOTS PERSPECTIVE

MARTH JANE "JENNIE" EBLEN

As a child, whenever I blew out a birthday candle, found a four leaf clover, or saw a falling star, I always wished, without hesitation, "Let there be world peace." Perhaps this wish is naive; the idea is a cliché to many. As a wish of innocence, it is fundamental to my vision of an ideal world, and I have no shame in claiming it. World Peace is still my wish.

I became involved in Peace Links through the same strategy that successfully reached thousands of women across our country—a Peace Links Tea. In the summer of 1984, I attended a tea sponsored by Peace Links North Carolina (PLNC) at the home of my young son's preschool teacher. I was thirty years old, a stay-at-home mom of two young children, and was completing my MA in anthropology at the University of Tennessee, Knoxville. My memory is that a group of mothers sat on the screened porch of the school, drank tea, ate goodies, and watched our children play in the preschool's playground. Isabel, our hostess, and Kim Hayes, then PLNC's Steering Committee coordinator, talked about Betty Bumpers's efforts and handed out information about this relatively new movement. In the relaxed and encouraging environment, we shared stories of apprehension about the threat of nuclear war.

The small group of mothers spoke of similar fears amid the summertime laughter of their children. Because of Betty's tale about how daughter Brooke inspired her to start Peace Links, these stories became known as our "Brooke stories." I vividly recall my Brooke story. In 1980, I sat in the hospital holding my ill son, overwhelmed by feelings of the need to protect him. Even though at that time my son was extremely ill with a rare bone infection, antibiotics could control it, and he would survive. What I feared most was that the world powers were threatening his future safety and existence with the nuclear arms race. I also felt a huge sense of desperation that I had no control of this nuclear insanity. As simple as it may seem, Peace Links succeeded by gathering women together in comfortable settings, letting them share their stories, and offering a vehicle to turn anxiety into action. Peace Links motivated women to share their concerns and stand up against the nuclear arms race. I was inspired to sign up, and within weeks I was called on to volunteer at the upcoming Peace Day event.

That fall, I helped with Peace Day 1984: A Family Festival of Peace. Hosting an annual Peace Day on the first Sunday of October was a nationwide Peace Links initiative. I helped set up and run the Peace Links booth, which gave out materials and sold event T-shirts. I was awed at this well-attended event that proved there were many community members with like-minded concerns for peace. A few months later, I was asked to join the PLNC Steering Committee and serve as the committee's secretary. As a new member of this volunteer committee, I was slightly intimidated and very quiet. I took meeting minutes to the best of my ability, but I did not understand all the information and jargon and was too unsure of myself to ask questions. For the first few meetings, I would not read my minutes aloud but instead handed them over for others to read. Over time, with the support of the other members, I became more confident and took a much more active role on the committee. Within four years, I was the PLNC Steering Committee coordinator.

From 1989 through 1991, I served as coordinator. Under my leadership, we actively participated in advocating for the Comprehensive Test Ban Treaty and took trips to Oak Ridge to protest the Y-12 nuclear production plant. I also gave a great deal of time to our Peace Day events: a Peace Child production in 1989 and Lightfest: Celebration of Peace & Hope in 1990. I coordinated, on behalf of PLNC, Asheville's Twentieth Anniversary Earth Day Parade and distributed Peace Links Worldwide Soviet Peace Pal Project letters among our community. For nine years, I volunteered for PLNC and believed that this service was my small contribution in helping to make the world safer for my children's generation.

Throughout my Peace Links career, I was able to meet and work with Betty five times. When she came to Asheville, she always created a buzz, but it was her friendliness, humility, and determination that made an impression on me. She was a master of networking—figuring out who needed to work with each other in order to make things happen. Betty would share humorous stories about her life, from her activist experiences to her grandchildren's antics. She kept PLNC updated with national and international political trends. It was always fascinating to hear a Washington insider's perspective on current activities. Most importantly, Betty served as a mentor, guiding us in our leadership of PLNC and continually inspiring PLNC members to carry on our efforts in peacemaking.

PLNC was one of the first regional Peace Links groups to be formed, and it developed into one of the most active and longest-lasting chapters. In 1983, it was cofounded by two dynamic women: Ginny Calloway and Becky Garlic. Becky rose to fame in the Peace Links movement by being featured with Betty Bumpers in *Parade* magazine (March 2, 1986). These founding co-coordinators of PLNC had the charisma to establish the chapter and make a significant impact both locally and nationally. By the time I became involved with the PLNC Steering Committee in 1985, leadership had passed to Kim Hayes.

An outside observer may have been surprised to know that PLNC did not represent all of North Carolina but served only a few western North Carolina counties surrounding Buncombe County and its county seat, Asheville. PLNC was just a small core group of between six and twelve volunteers, called the Steering Committee, who carried out all the activities of the organization for seventeen years. While PLNC had 501(c)3 status, it was not a typical nonprofit organization because there was no paid staff or office facility. We had an annual budget averaging less than $5,000. One of our founding members, Kitty Boniske, bought and renovated a historic house in the Montford area of Asheville and created the Center for New Priorities, offered as a free meeting space to a variety of local groups, including PLNC.

Generally, Peace Links regional chapters were autonomous organizations with their own organizational structure and homegrown projects and events. PLNC did not often interact with other regional chapters but did maintain a very significant relationship with Peace Links Worldwide (PLW). PLW, the national central office located in Washington, D.C., was very supportive of the local chapters. Even though PLW had excellent paid staff and a governance board, most of us considered it "Betty's headquarters," for she was the face of the Peace Links movement. PLW provided local chapters with informational brochures about the arms race, marketing materials, packets on how to conduct activities (such as Peace Panels, Coffee Parties, and Women's Forums), and information on how to be successful activists. Being affiliated with PLW and using the Peace Links brand did not require a membership fee. At first, each chapter was asked to submit quarterly reports of activities and number of participants, but accountability to the national office became very informal. One requirement from PLW was nonpartisanship, which Betty considered a key strategy and strength of Peace Links.

As PLNC evolved, we found it most efficient to promote awareness of the nuclear arms race through annual Peace Day community events. The first year I was involved, we undertook a remarkable project for Peace Day. Betty had been cultivating relationships with women in the USSR and realized that American and Soviet women shared anxiety about the buildup of nuclear weapons. In 1985, PLW coordinated the first Soviet Women's Exchange, bringing fifteen Soviet women to visit fourteen U.S. cities. Our Peace Links chapter was selected as one of the host sites. Concerning this nationwide project, Betty was quoted in the Asheville paper:

> We've worked very hard for the day when we can welcome Soviet women as our guests. What is critically important is that they will see us—ordinary American citizens—as we really are in all our diversity. And when they return to the Soviet Union, I hope they and we will know that even though we are separated by a physical gulf of thousands of miles and an emotional gulf of enormously different ideas and histories, we do have—as women and mothers—the same hopes, fears and dreams for ourselves and our children.[17]

Truthfully, our small, newly developed Steering Committee was stunned and a bit intimidated about being selected as a host community, but we plunged ahead with planning for the visit. A few months before the women were to arrive, we learned that Soviet citizens were not allowed to come to Asheville (we believe this was because Asheville was home to the National Climatic Data Center). By that time, we had made elaborate preparations for the Soviet visitor. To our relief, local and federal government leaders acted on our behalf and got approval for the visit. From October 22 to 23, we hosted Margrita Ziborova, Yekaterina Orlova, and Molohat Shahobova, accompanied by Elinor Bedell, a congressional Peace Link. We planned an itinerary that included a wide variety of local attractions from a tour of the Biltmore Estate to a visit to the Vance birthplace, a community concert, receptions, and meals in Peace Link members' homes. All of this was a whirlwind of exciting activities, but the most thrilling part for me, a young mom awed by the very accomplished Soviet women, was having them in my humble home for a meal.

It may be hard to imagine now, but this was such a groundbreaking effort. In 1985, our countries were still in the midst of the Cold War, and our group of everyday American women was breaking through many national policies and preconceived ideas concerning our imagined "enemies." A meaningful moment was when we took the Soviet visitors to the airport and exchanged emotional hugs and warm blessings. Even though we could not understand each other's words, there was no doubt that we were linked in friendship and the wish for peace between our countries. Betty's vision for this exchange had come true! In the next ten years, PLNC participated in at least five other Soviet Women's Exchanges.

Another significant local accomplishment that was spearheaded by PLW in the early 1990s was the Peace Pal Project, which offered women in the USSR the opportunity to have a pen pal with women in the USA. This project addressed one of Betty's strategies for peace: to build relationships between women around the world. The response from Soviet citizens was overwhelming, much more than anyone at PLW had anticipated. One way PLW facilitated finding pen pals for the thousands of Soviets that responded to the Peace Pal Project newspaper add was to send a large stack of letters from the USSR to each regional Peace Links chapter. PLNC distributed hundreds of letters seeking pen pals throughout our community.

Betty's vision for this project was realized when my friend Helen Dezendorf began writing an English teacher named Galina, who lived in Verkhnaya Salda in the Ural Mountains about 900 miles east of Moscow. Today, Helen and Galina remain great friends and have been able to share in each other's lives for the past twenty years! Now they can communicate more easily by the Internet and phone. Helen has visited Galina in Russia four times.[18]

Looking back now, I am amazed at the significant impact that PLNC made in our local community as well as nationally and worldwide. The fact that this influential organization was completely volunteer driven makes the organization's accomplishments even more impressive, validates Betty's model for community organizing, and recognizes the dedication of the volunteers. Along with the vital support and guidance of Betty and the national organization, PLNC was able to sustain itself for over seventeen years as an active, volunteer organization for several reasons: (1) Peace Links participants were connected by their shared beliefs and a focused mission against nuclear war and promoting peace. (2) Betty's core strategy of networking and building community partnerships accelerated the spread of the message to many diverse community members. (3) The mostly female group valued relationship building and created an environment that nurtured leaders. PLNC's leaders not only contributed to the success of the organization but also continued to share their leadership skills, specifically in the realm of nonprofit management and advocacy, and have made a positive difference in their communities.

From her many years of experience with community organizing, Betty brought her wisdom of working with established agencies and organizations. PLW partnered with many other national peace and social justice organizations and encouraged the local chapters to do the same. A key message from Betty to the regional chapters was to recognize the strength of local like-minded groups and to incorporate their expertise and networks to further the goals of Peace Links. Understanding this concept of intentional coalition building, PLNC collaborated extensively with many local entities, including Physicians for Social Responsibility, the Women's International League for Peace and Freedom, the League of Women Voters, SANE, the YWCA, Sister Cities, Educators for Social Responsibility, the WNC United Nations Association, and Ecumenical Peacemakers. PLNC was deliberate in organizing Peace Day events that would include the arts community, educators, environmental groups, college students, and faith groups so that their base of influence could expand beyond peace activists. The PLNC Steering Committee became knowledgeable in many types of advocacy from education to lobbying. Members learned how to efficiently collaborate with the media and local, state, and federal policymakers.

As PLNC's influence continued to grow, it often led the local peace movement and other groups sought out PLNC to join in their events and projects. In fact, I first met Betty when she came to our community as a keynote speaker for the New Priorities Conference in September 1987. This two-day conference on peace, social justice, and environmental issues was a model for coalition building—over forty organizations supported or participated in this event. I greatly anticipated meeting Betty and was surprised to find how down to earth she was. At this event, Betty was motivational in her straightforward and heartfelt remarks, although she was not an exceptional speaker. North Carolinians could relate to her Southern accent, colloquialisms, and familiar stories. The fact that her stage presence was personable rather than elitist was one of her most appealing characteristics. Betty came across as an everyday person, a role model who made us feel we could also become leaders and make a difference in bringing peace to the world.

Betty exemplified a powerful, influential female leader, and the PLNC Steering Committee nurtured female leadership. Steering Committee members supported, encouraged, and sincerely appreciated each other. Members took the time to become good friends, united in our work. Each brought unique experiences and skills to the group, and by working closely together, we shared and taught one another. Linda McLean verified this: "When I look back at what we accomplished, especially in the variety and quality of our annual Peace Day events, I see the gifts of each coordinator shining through . . . it was hands-on learning and shared leadership. Our little Peace Links group was a safe nest for learning how to lead and collaborate."[19]

Throughout the years, all Peace Links Steering Committee participants had opportunities to learn effective nonprofit management skills. As we promoted peace, we also learned how to facilitate meetings, create agendas, give speeches, create marketing plans, write press releases, resolve conflict, raise funds, negotiate contracts, and manage volunteers. We became experts in event planning as we coordinated annual community-wide Peace Day events.

My Peace Links experience was a very valuable part of my personal growth and education. It was a perfect model for service learning with meaningful community service that taught about civic responsibility and strengthening community. My initiation into community service with a wise, nurturing female group greatly affected my leadership style of inclusiveness and encouragement. When I first became involved with PLNC, I was a young woman who did not feel comfortable reading aloud her own meeting minutes. Recently, I've received community awards and heard that people respect my work as a leader, albeit a somewhat tenacious activist who chairs numerous nonprofit boards, happily speaks at community events, and corners politicians to advocate for children.

Betty Bumpers and Peace Links helped empower a group of women across our country to value relationship building, collaboration, determination, and dedication to the vision of peace. In addition to increasing awareness of nuclear war issues, one of the most valuable outcomes of Betty's Peace Links movement was the creation of knowledgeable, skilled female community leaders.

PEACE LINKS ARKANSAS

MARGARET WHILLOCK[20]

MW: [In response to questions about her involvements with Peace Links] In 1984, I was the executive director of Peace Links, Arkansas. I had heard Betty speak in Little Rock. There was lots of publicity about it, and I had friends who were involved in it. Betty and I probably met first at a political event. My husband, Carl, had worked for federal congressman Jim Trimble for eight years when he was a young man. Carl came from a long line of yellow dog Democrats. Congressman Trimble was the Democratic representative from the western district.

BB: We knew him from his campaigns because he was our representative. I voted for him, but I was busy with my kids.

MW: [In response to a question about Peace Links activities] We had Peace Day, and we had a breakfast at the Medical Center for doctors. Betty brought in Howard Hiatt from Harvard in the fall. We also went to smaller towns and put on seminars, participated in fairs, we even had several chapters of Peace Links in high schools—if Betty was in town, she spoke. We encouraged the people at our meetings to ask questions. It was controversial. One of my children said, "My mother is going to get mugged." Somebody wrote a play [*Peace Child*] about children and peace, and I knew people at the Arts Center who let us put on the play there. Naturally, there was advertising about the play, and a group began to picket the Arkansas Arts Center. They called us communists and got the local TV stations to come out as well as the other press. We got a better audience after that and had four performances. One lesson I learned while working for Peace Links was how many people are afraid of the idea of world peace. This seems to be true today, I am sorry to say.

Betty was the draw, the attraction for Peace Links. She expressed what many women thought privately. Everybody knew about her, and everybody wanted to meet her. Betty has received numerous honors and awards over the years. The University of Arkansas and Hendrix gave her an honorary doctorate. If Betty had lived in another day and age, she would have run a Fortune 500 company. She is creative and innovative. People identify her with the immunization program, and the beauty of that program and Peace Links was that they empowered women. She trusted women to run those, and then she let them do their thing.

People from all across the country met the Soviet women when they came to visit. A group of us went to Washington. I especially remember the woman who spoke about the siege of Leningrad during the war. As a child, she lived through the siege, but her little sister and mom and dad died. She felt lucky to have survived. She told us, "One of the highlights of my childhood was when American schoolchildren sent us a box with gum and little treats."

BB: Then we also worked with Pamela Harriman. Her husband was an ambassador under FDR and the secretary of commerce for Truman. She was ambassador to France. Harriman loved the idea that we used in-place organizations. Sometimes, I would be seated with him at dinners and things because, although he was hard of hearing, he could hear my voice.

MW: [Pamela Harriman's] help was worth having, and she was interested in Peace Links.

BB: In 1985, we had fifteen or sixteen Soviet women accompanied by one or two Senate women.

MW: You brought in smaller groups of Soviet women. Their own people wouldn't let them come in. Even now, Russians can't travel the way we can.

BB: Another big place that was very active with Peace Links was Pennsylvania. The wife of the president of the University of Pennsylvania was active. Just last year, the Pennsylvania Peace Links quit and gave the copyrighted name to someone else. The archives were boxed up and went to the University of Pittsburgh.

MW: The *Arkansas Democrat* used to give Peace Links good coverage.

BB: The greatest contribution of Peace Links was that we prepared this country for accepting the former Soviets. When the women came, we woodshedded them in D.C. for three days and told them not to talk about the military and the fact of the wall. We put them all over the country in open forums. They talked about the workplace, education, and health care. People realized they were people just like us. They were mothers and fathers who wanted exactly the same things as us for their children.

MW: [When I worked at the Clinton White House] I remember when Betty brought a bunch of Methodist bishops to the White House. Betty wandered off, and the Secret Service came looking for me and said, "You're missing one." Betty was resting in a hall somewhere.

One of the most enjoyable things was traveling with Betty. We had the satisfaction of accomplishing something. We were following the mode of our Methodist upbringing. [In response about difficulties of Peace Links] There was a lot of controversy. Some men were making fun of it; they might not argue, but they'd say a sort of ho, ho. Other men were very angry about it.

BB: Men didn't get it. Peace Links challenged their attitude that you resolve problems with conflict. We can't afford wars—that hasn't even changed. They make this new generation of nuclear weapons and think they'll solve things.

MW: Macho mentality.

BB: Civilization won't make another step forward until women all over the world get their rights.

NOTES

1. Betty Bumpers, "Article for *Unitarian Universalist World*," manuscript, July 7, 1986, Peace Links Records Addendum (MC 907a), series 1, subseries 4, box 7, folder 7-10, Special Collections, University of Arkansas Libraries, Fayetteville, 6–7.
2. Materials within quotation marks are from Bumpers's speeches or writings, cited as endnotes below. Materials outside quotation marks are derived from interviews with Betty Bumpers by Anna and Jennie Eblen, August 29–31, 2005; May 14, 2006; October 2–6, 2007; and February 24–26, 2009.
3. Bumpers, "Article for *Unitarian Universalist World*," 1.
4. Bumpers, "Article for *Unitarian Universalist World*," 2.
5. Betty Bumpers, "I've Spent the Past Two Years," speech manuscript (n.d.), Peace Links Records Addendum (MC 907a), series 1, subseries 4, box 7, folder 7-10, Special Collections, University of Arkansas Libraries, Fayetteville, 1–2.
6. Bumpers, "Article for *Unitarian Universalist World*," 2–3. Verb tense has some changes from present, present perfect, and future tense in the original to past tense in this chapter for citations of this speech.
7. Betty Bumpers, "Ship of State," speech manuscript, WAND conference (n.d.), Peace Links Records Addendum (MC 907a), series 1, subseries 4, box 7, folder 7-10, Special Collections, University of Arkansas Libraries, Fayetteville, 4. Verb tense has some changes from present, present perfect, and future tense in the original to past tense in this chapter for citations of this speech.
8. Bumpers, "I've Spent the Past Two Years," 1.
9. Betty Bumpers, "Making Our Voices Heard," speech manuscript, WAND conference (n.d.), Peace Links Records Addendum (MC 907a), series 1, subseries 4, box 7, folder 7-10, Special Collections, University of Arkansas Libraries, Fayetteville, 1. Verb tense has some changes from present, present perfect, and future tense in the original to past tense in this chapter for citations of this speech.
10. Betty Bumpers, "Wilton Peace Award Speech," manuscript, March 27, 1986 Peace Links Records Addendum (MC 907a), series 1, subseries 4, box 7, folder 7-9, Special Collections, University of Arkansas Libraries, Fayetteville, 1–3. Verb tense has some changes from present, present perfect, and future tense in the original to past tense in this chapter for citations of this speech.
11. Bumpers, "Wilton Peace Award Speech," 2.
12. Bumpers, "Article for *Unitarian Universalist World*," 9.
13. Bumpers, "I've Spent the Past Two Years," 2.
14. Bumpers, "Wilton Peace Award Speech," paraphrased from final paragraph, 2.
15. Bumpers, "Wilton Peace Award Speech," 3.
16. Bumpers, "I've Spent the Past Two Years," 3, 4.
17. *Asheville Citizen*, October 6, 1985.

18. Helen Dezendorf, interview by Jennie Eblen, May 2009.
19. Linda McLean, interview by Jennie Eblen, May 2009.
20. Margaret Whillock (MW) and Betty Bumpers (BB), February 26, 2009, field notes from interview by Anna Eblen and Jennie Eblen, Fayetteville, Arkansas. Margaret Whillock, BSE, University of Arkansas, taught school, served as deputy director of the Clinton's White House Visitor's Office, and volunteered extensively. On December 5, 2009, interview details were corrected by Whillock.

II

Developing as an Activist

FOUR

Family and Neighbors Survive the Great Depression

Being raised by a father who needed four boys in the farm business instead of three girls and one boy, we all worked like men. He always convinced us that we could do anything we wanted to do in this world, if we worked hard enough.

CONVERSATIONS WITH BETTY

"I grew up on a farm in Arkansas, blessed by an eighth-grade-educated father and a mother with three semesters in a small college—both very commonsensical, devoted parents. It was the era of the Great Depression. Neighbors looked after neighbors. And our food, which we grew, was shared with those who were in poverty and had none. We did our best to honor the teachings of our Sunday school teachers at the one-room Methodist church, which, along with a one-room grade school, were the only community buildings in Grand Prairie, Arkansas. It was six miles from Charleston, population 851, where my future husband Dale Bumpers was growing up in only slightly better conditions."[1]

My older brother and sister went to that rural schoolhouse in Grand Prairie. Their school did not have buses, and I remember the two of them on one horse, riding to get there. Later, I started first grade in a little town called Branch, where my grandparents Callan lived. In my second-grade year, the rural schools were consolidated, and I rode a school bus to Charleston. A huge area had consolidated to build County Line School. As part of the consolidation, people in the area had to provide a road and keep it in good condition for the bus to run on. My dad worked digging ditches and putting that dirt down on the road. He had a kind of scoop that we called a slip, with two handles on it, and he would hitch that up to our team of mules. Think how laborious that was—miles and miles of county road. But people in the community, all the men and able-bodied family members, were glad to help maintain those roads, to pack down dirt and the gravel the county gave us.

Our bus didn't have a heater in it, just an old wooden floor, and it would be chilly. We were the first kids picked up, so we had the longest ride and would get so cold. My dad got these big flat stones about an inch thick and put them in our oven early in the morning. Then he would take them out and put them on the floor of the bus where we could put our feet on them. We'd try to share the rocks with as many of the kids as we could. I remember my older brother getting into kind of a fight with some big bully kid who tried to push our feet off of it. He wanted to get his feet on there and hog the warm rock, but my brother took him on.

Another time, we were on the monkey row—that's a row in the center of the bus, not the benches along the sides. The monkey row had a long stool, not very wide, that we straddled, with other kids behind and in front of us. One time a boy got in there with his gang and tried to shove and put us in a sandwich; they could squeeze a person to death. My brother, who was very protective of his three younger sisters, told the boy not to hurt us. The boy said he didn't care if he hurt us or not, and my brother got into a scuffle, threatening to knock his head off, and there's no telling what could have happened.

My brother was the apple of my mother's eye, and she relied on him to look after us. He was her oldest, and I never felt like he was the favorite child or anything, but we just knew that she relied on him a lot. They had a very close relationship. He helped take care of us because my mother had had a child about every two years until she had the four of us. You can imagine how much she depended on him as the oldest one, with our living out on a farm and my dad traveling. My brother herded us around like an old shepherd dog, even at school.

The girls had to wear long underwear to school in the wintertime with big, long stockings hitched up by suspenders. We'd get hot in the daytime, and sometimes our stockings unhitched and rolled down. We would have this big roll of underwear up here at our waists and big rolls of stockings down here at our ankles. And, oh, we were an embarrassment for him. My brother would catch us on the playground, pull up the stockings, hitch them, and roll down the underwear. Other rural girls wore the same things, but I'd be embarrassed by my lumpy stockings when they fell down.

At school I didn't have a favorite subject. I was no good at math or spelling, but I was kind of interested in history. I can remember having to learn all the days of the week and the months in the year and how to spell them, and I had a fifth-grade teacher who taught us the Twenty-Third Psalm and the Lord's Prayer. She would sometimes send us out on the playground, where there was a big, wonderful tree. Once I drew a skeletal tree, and she put it up in our classroom. From then on, I fancied myself an artist.

At recess, we played all sorts of games, like jump rope and hopscotch, on the playground with a group of friends. Other times, we'd form a long line and go around and try to sling the end one off, like a whip. We had little posts that went all the way around the perimeter of our playground, and one great skill was jumping from one of those posts to the other. I still have a deep scar as the result of that. My foot slipped on the corner of that post. It bruised the bone, and I think maybe I had that bone infection people get.

I enjoyed school, of course, but I was a daydreamer. I suffered from narcolepsy—not severe—but I had it. I'd sit still, and I had episodes of sleep that I couldn't control. I would get sleepy and just zone out; it happened a lot growing up. My mother said my brother and I were the night owls. We would stay up all night or go to bed early and then wake up really early. My dad would get me up to do homework early in the morning instead of at night because that was my best time to learn.

School was a happy time, and I have fond memories. We had to take our lunch because we didn't have such a thing as a cafeteria. We always had meat of some kind: sausage or sliced bacon or side meat. My mother was always making fudge or some candy out of sugar and water, so there was a piece of candy for dessert. She'd pack fried chicken from breakfast or even quail, as we had lots of quail. This was during the Depression, and some of the girls who lived in town were eager to trade lunches with me. When I think about it, they had store-bought bread, which we called lightening bread or light bread, and sandwich spread when it first came out. The sandwich spread was just mayonnaise with some pickles. Oh, I thought that was wonderful on light bread, but what the girls wanted was the meat in my lunch.

For the first twelve years of my life, we lived out in the country. My parents moved to the Flanagan farmland after they were married, and my grandfather Callan helped them build a house. We lived in this six-room frame house, with a screened-in back porch, about a quarter mile away from my dad's parents. Family lived all around; an uncle and aunt and their kids lived nearby.

I'm the middle Flanagan child, with an older brother, Callans; an older sister, Maggie; and a younger sister, Ruth. We were four active kids living in six rooms. My parents had a bedroom, and there were two beds in each bedroom. My brother slept out in the screened-in back porch a lot of the time, except in extremely cold weather. After we built an extra room with an attic over the storm cellar, he took over the attic for his room.

Our house had a deep front porch. We'd take some mattresses and sleep out there in the hot summertime or sleep out in the yard, trying to get cool air. Past the front porch, you entered what we called the living room. Mother had a piano, which she played, and a few occasional chairs and tables in there. Next to that was the dining room, which was about the same size and had a potbelly stove in one corner.

In that room, mother stored the quilting frame, and she'd have a quilt up on this wooden frame, suspended by wires attached to screws in the ceiling. We wrapped the ropes around carriers when she wanted to bring it down. We had to put it back up when we were finished because it was right over the dining table, which was a long table with benches. She'd always have a quilt up in our house. In the summer, we'd play, then come in and quilt. When we got home from school, she would feed us or have something for us to eat, maybe a cookie. Lots of times in the winter, if it was cold, she'd have supper early because we'd be chilled. After we finished our chores or between when we got off school and ate supper, we would sit in that room with the big, old potbelly stove. She'd let the quilt down, and we'd all sit around it, talking about our day's activities and quilting until bedtime. My brother was an excellent quilter, but we never did break Ruth into quilting; she never did learn to sew.

Past that room was the kitchen with a great wood cook stove, thanks to our grandfather, I'm sure. It had a hot water well in it and a warming oven up behind, as wide as the stove, and that is where my mother would keep food warm. She would put a bowl of peas or potatoes, left from our big meal at noon, up in the kitchen cabinets. Then we'd have the cold vegetables with a hot pan of cornbread she had made just for dinner.

We ate a big breakfast, then a very big noon meal, and then we just had warmed-over food in the evening. Along with the hot cornbread and leftover cold vegetables, we always had dried fruit. Three things were always on our table: stewed dried fruit, molasses, and hot bread or hot rolls of some kind. We mixed the molasses with butter to put on the cornbread. I still like to eat cooked vegetables cold.

The Snow family lived nearby, and I'm sure he was English because they had an English garden that I think about to this day. He and his wife grew gooseberries, sunflowers, and vegetables, and they had a wonderful orchard. They lived down the hill and had a well with a springhouse that kept water cool. We lived up on top of the hill, so we didn't have a springhouse.

His place was near a road where some public conveyance went through daily, and his buggy shed was right on the road. He did repairs on other people's buggies and wagons. Their house was a log cabin with a front porch and a great big room that had a big fireplace. That big room was where they sat and where they slept; there were two beds in it. A lean-to in the back had another bedroom. The long kitchen had a table where they ate and where Ma Snow cooked. Some steps led down into the backyard, and they kept their yard scraped. Two or three old cedar trees were trimmed up high, and it was cool. I liked being on that front porch, out in that cool yard, and in that English garden.

Most of all, we loved to get into their living room. The only way in was to come out on the little porch and go in through two other front doors. It was the ultimate for us, getting into that room, where they had an organ and a big dictionary on top of a table. The few times that I was allowed in there to go through the dictionary and look at the pictures of animals in Africa, I was thrilled. I was fascinated by the animals, especially African animals, so looking through that dictionary was a big treat. I also read every one of the books in the school library about animals and adventures in Africa. Above the dictionary table was the calendar. I don't know what vintage it was, but the women pictured had to have been early twentieth century. There was a woman with a cigarette in her mouth and a 1920s dress dancing down this trail with a lot of cocktail glasses and liquor. And on the other side was a lady at church. I don't know what she was doing, but she was on her way to heaven. Mainly, I just remember seeing the wicked side. One of them was funneled into heaven, and the one on the other side was funneled into hell. We would talk about that picture.

Our backyard and our neighbors' backyards were scraped—we scraped everything down with a hoe. It was just packed dirt. We didn't scrape our front yard, but it wasn't mowed unless my dad ran through it once or twice with the big hay mower, which would cut it down low. We also pulled the grass when we were on the farm—I don't remember having a lawn mower.

We had a big garden, and I remember the hills of dirt mounded up for burying carrots and cabbage. In the early part of winter, I had to go out in the cold and dig out carrots or other things; I don't think they lasted all winter. Then I would get canned or stored stuff from the storm cellar, and we'd serve that. It was as self-sufficient as you can get.

It was rough, back in those days in Arkansas, during the Depression. My dad tried all kinds of things because he had four kids to feed. He tried making molasses, using our sorghum. He had a cane press, and other people brought their cane to us for pressing. During Dust Bowl times, we'd get some dust storms, and once I was shocked to see the wagon wheels up to their hubs in dust, it was so dry. At the press, a mule would go around and around, and we kids fed the cane into the press. The juice would be put into pan and cooked it until it turned into molasses. They had to keep a fire under it and stir it with a big paddle. People would share what was produced, and the process went on for days and weeks. This wasn't done often, and we didn't raise sorghum for very long—maybe it was too dry there. My dad did it as an experiment, to earn money to feed us.

It was a different era, growing up on a farm—a really rural farm, in a rural area. We never knew we were poor. We were, of course—everybody was kind of poor. But we never had a poverty mentality. We knew people who left—we had an uncle and aunt who went to California with their four kids in that migration out of the Dust Bowl.

I remember hobos coming through, and my mother always tried to find something to feed them. We didn't have a lot, but we'd have something to give, and sometimes they'd work for a few days to help dad out. We had a smokehouse behind the house, and my brother would trap muskrats, raccoons, and possums; skin them; and tack the skins up there. He sold those some, even when he was young. He and our dad also hunted game for us to eat.

Being raised by a father who needed four boys instead of three girls and one boy because his business was farming, we all worked like men. He just treated all of us like we were men; he threw the world at us, and we didn't know anything else but to try to carry it. We just did anything and everything. He always convinced us that we could do anything we wanted to do in this world if we worked hard enough. We took on jobs because he needed sons on the farm. I remember mother hitching a rope around me or around two of us, and we would pull the plow while she plowed the garden. And I mean, we worked.

One of my favorite pictures of my dad shows a cocky young man courting my mother, sitting in a buggy with his leg crossed. It was so typical of him. I talk like my dad; I picked up a lot of my way of talking from being from the South and from my father, who was a smart man even though he only had an eighth-grade education. He would substitute words and expressions for his lack of vocabulary. One time, he was asking my husband about a well-known politician who'd just been elected in Arkansas. Dale was trying to explain to my dad that the politician was a fine man who did a lot of good, but Dale didn't include much criticism. My dad said, "Well, I've seldom seen a bird whose feathers all lie in one direction." You know, that communicates to everybody.

Another time, when my dad was asked his opinion about someone, he said, "Well, I just think he's caught a horse that's too tall for him to reach up and bridle." People understand, and I've used a lot of that kind of language, too. So many people can relate to that kind of language who can't if you use a regular vocabulary. It's amazing, and that's still true in this country.

My dad was also an observant man. He told me this story, and I think it's priceless. It also tells you where I get my liberal views, and it tells you more about colloquialisms and the ability to communicate. My dad never referred to the people who came down there and bought up land for taxes except to say, "They ain't anything but goddamn Yankees." Or he called them carpetbaggers.[2]

I knew every carpetbagger family who'd come and bought land, and by then, it was their second or third generation. One carpetbagger family owned this little country store that had a cotton gin. During the early WPA [the New Deal's Work Progress Administration] days, we'd go by the store in the wagon. We tried to raise at least one bale of cotton every year to buy our school clothes. We hoped to maybe get two bales, but the land was worn out by this time.

My dad passed by that store, and there was the old man who owned it. The store still had three generations working in it, and the old man was just fretting and fuming and cussing anytime and every time my dad went in there. He fussed, "The goddamn WPA's using my taxes for something useless, some worthless program."

My dad said, "Well, it's helping all of us."

"Oh, it is not; it's doing nothing but spending my tax dollars and blah, blah."

My dad said, "Yeah, it's helping all of us. Most of the time when I used to come by here, you and junior were sitting out on the west end of the store in the shade, whittling and spitting. When I'd come back in the afternoon from road building, you'd be sitting on the other end in the shade, leaning back, whittling, and spitting. Now, you're inside waiting on people. Yeah, it's helping all of us."

My dad told another story about the same man. When Dad was a lad, about fifteen, hunting was the big thing. My dad had a shotgun, and we had lots of quail down there. He'd hunt them, then gut the birds and nail them up on the side of the smokehouse to dry them out. When he had a number of them, he'd sack them up, take them down to that store, and sell them to that old man.

Dad said, "The first time I ever remember being disrespectful to one of my elders, I'd taken my sack of quail down there. I'd stack them up on the counter, and he'd pick one up, and he'd sniff. Then he'd put it down over here and pick another one up and sniff and put it down over here, then pick another one up and sniff and set it down over there. These over here were good, and those over there were bad.

"Then the old man said, 'Well.' He'd get through the sack sniffing and stacking, and he'd give me two cents or a nickel for the good ones. About the other stack, he'd say, 'I'll feed them to my dogs.' And he'd just pull them off the counter, and they'd drop down in the trash can."

"By God, the second time I took my sack of quail in there, when he was done stacking them up, I put my hand on his 'bad' quail and said, 'My dog likes quail too.' You know, I knew he was cheating me. Even if the quail were bad, which they weren't, I knew he was cheating me because sometimes I took them back. I'd mix them in with the next batch I took down, and then he'd take most of them."

We knew exactly how our family felt about everybody in the community. We'd listen, and we'd know they were either "an honest man" and "I'd crawl in the trenches with him" or "she's a fine woman." Or they were "thieving sons of bitches" or "he's a you-know." We heard my parents' attitudes about almost everybody and knew their sense of what everyone was about. I knew if neighbors were good guys or if they were bad because my mom and dad talked to each other all the time.

One day later in my life, my dad and Dale were talking about a gentleman who was one of these very posh, real Southern gentlemen, and he and his wife had a disabled child. His wife was very pretty and genteel, and she wasn't about to take care of a handicapped child. She had been raised like her mother, who probably had owned slaves. The wife just wouldn't take responsibility, but she was pretty, and she was charming. That man never, ever worked, but he was a handsome, sweet, dear man.

One day, Dale asked my dad, "Babe, what did that gentleman ever do to make a living? I don't remember him ever making a living or ever working or anything." And my dad said, "Well, my God, son, he never struck a lick of work, after the first Red Cross flour came to town." My dad was talking about when the WPA started giving out commodities like Red Cross flour—it was sort of like welfare, but I don't think they called it that. He meant that the man got commodities for his food and some money for his disabled child and didn't work after that. The gentleman had other children who worked, and they probably helped him out.

My parents believed that kids need to know those things. They do need to—that's valuable information passed on to kids. It's not tacky, you know; it's just reality. It's important to understand what it means to say, "He never did a lick of work since the first Red Cross flour came to town." We knew my dad's idea that the gentleman counted on help that came from the government or from the state. My dad thought the gentleman owned his home, and it just didn't cost him much money to live. Maybe he did some kind of work my dad didn't know about.

Dad couldn't stand our school bus driver. The driver was an old man out of Charleston, and he wouldn't sweep out the bus to keep it clean. One morning, dad took a broom and said, "By God, I want you to sweep that bus out. You are either going to take this broom and sweep it out, or I am going to sweep it out with you." So the driver swept the bus out.

That is just the kind of man my dad was, a fiery little Irishman who wasn't about to put up with a bus so dirty that we would come home from school in the summertime hot and sweaty with dust mustaches. When the bus bounced, the dust inside would poof up and get all over us. Sometimes, the driver wouldn't put the windows down, and I remember my dad telling my brother, "Ask him to lower the windows so you children can get some air. And by God, if he won't lower them, knock one of them out." And my brother did it. Yeah, he sure did; he knocked out a window. The driver wanted to confront my dad and huff, but he didn't dare because my dad would have told him to take a skyrocket to the moon.

My dad wasn't a bully; he was just a sensible man, and he wasn't about to put up with a driver abusing the kids. Dad would say, "By God, we pay your salary. We're the parents whose kids you haul around, and there's no sense in you treating them like this." And so he straightened that driver up pretty good.

I remember helping my dad build levees to stop erosion on the land. He would plow along a line of little red flags the Extension Service had put out to help him prevent erosion. The Agriculture Extension people also taught us how to use poison in our gardens to stop potato bugs. We used to go up and down our potato rows picking the bugs off and dropping them in a can, a little bucket of kerosene. The Extension agents taught us how to sprinkle powders, among other things. The first home-canning demonstrations were put on by the Service's home economists; all of this happened during President Franklin Roosevelt's administration.

My dad had a big truck we used to take green beans or peas or things like that into the community kitchen for canning on a particular day of the month. Like everyone else, we shared what we brought. He always had a big garden; he thought a garden had to be a truck patch, so we'd have bushels of green beans to share. They'd do up a number of cans of green beans, and then everybody who had participated would share them. Other times, I can remember picking green beans very early in the morning; he'd take them in immediately to the cannery, and he would be paid for those. The Extension people came to those little communities. Our canning kitchen at Charleston was just a church and a building left from the rural school.

My dad raised beef because he loved meat, and he always had beef or a hog fattening. He didn't take the hogs in for canning because everyone could cure their own hams, but there's not an easy way to cure beef. The first time we had beef all year-round was when we took beef into that kitchen with its tin-can sealer. It was great, and Extension did that all over the country, especially the South.

My dad was a visionary about cattle trading. He started raising, then trading cattle when the farm was farmed out and there was no way to make money on it. We had, I would guess, 150 acres for crops and pasture, but he didn't much like dirt farming anyway. He would do some small cash crops, but he didn't particularly like that; he liked the selling and trading.

My dad made the effort to get back to the farm on a Sunday afternoon, even if he'd been away trading. When he'd come home at noon, we'd all take a nap lying down on the floor because it's cooler on the floor, you know. He'd be lying on the floor, and sometimes we'd wrestle or play games. We'd lie down there, and he'd just go to sleep, and we would use him as a pillow.

My mom was a smart woman and went to college for close to two years, working towards her teaching certificate. Then she fell in love with Babe, my dad. Her mother had died when she was five and her brother was two. My grandfather remarried when my mom was about seven or eight; I don't think he waited over three years to marry again. My mother was pretty spoiled because her father loved her and tried to take care of her.

My mother's family was Southern, and they owned some stores in the country and a larger store in Charleston, which was a pretty, thriving little town. She grew up working as the buyer in the department store there for her dad. She'd take a train into Fort Smith, about thirty miles away, to look at dry goods and do the buying for the store.

So she had studied and worked before getting married, but when she married and moved out on the farm with my dad, they had four kids—bing, bing, bing, bing. Back in those days, it was a chauvinistic society. My dad was a pretty strong-willed man. Mother was a hypochondriac, though I think she turned to illness as a way of getting attention. She had migraine headaches, but still she worked like mad, canning and doing all the housework; she didn't have a lazy bone in her body. My mother was a big woman, too. She was five feet nine inches and kind of large; she was bigger than any of the three daughters until she got osteoporosis in her late eighties.

Back in those days, women were taught homemaking skills really young. She had a wash pot going all the time so she could sterilize things. I remember several times scalding my fingers because we had to dry dishes, and she'd never let us touch one until she had poured boiling water over it. I'm sure the skills she had been taught helped to keep us from being sick. I don't remember missing school or having a sore throat. I'm sure we had some colds but not nearly as often as a lot of kids did. She used to say, "Just stay away from those sick kids—they've got those old green-snot colds." And she had one of the first washing machines, a little gasoline-powered one that went pop-pop-pop.

My mother was also a very clever seamstress. She would buy this pretty, flower-print calico cloth and make two or three little dresses with bloomers to match. She'd also make things out of flour and seed sacks—those cloth sacks came with colors back then.

We had dried fruit all winter long for nutrition. In the summertime, we would put out pieces of sheet iron, and we'd lay peaches, apples, and even grapes on them. My mother would put some kind of wire over the fruit and then worn-out muslin tea towels to keep the flies off. We'd put the sheets up on the roof over the screened-in porch to dry. If it rained, we'd have to run out to get them, and then we'd have to put them back up every morning. I especially remember drying peaches, and to this day I still have peach jam, and I love it.

Mother would wax our kitchen floor once a month or so because she wanted things clean. Of course, living out in the country, we didn't have much traffic, but with just the wind, there'd be dust. She would melt paraffin and mix it with—I think it was kerosene—then put it on a rag mop. After she'd waxed the floors, we'd play games to do the polishing, which was one of our chores. If we had old underwear or worn-out overalls, we'd take turns sitting on that and slinging each other around by the legs, polishing that floor. I remember getting a few knots on my head from being slung into the wall or something. Or we'd put things on our feet and skate all over. But we'd also have to get into the corners and around the edges of the walls.

My mother was a night person, and she never slept much. She was just a bed head in the mornings until ten or eleven o'clock. Of course, she had to get up at four o'clock because my dad was up, being a farmer, and she had to fix breakfast. She'd be kind of staggering around, half asleep. One time my dad fixed her a hot toddy. I remember we got up, and she was behind the stove, kind of giggling and scooting down the wall; dad was laughing and giggling, too. I'm sure that she was about half, well, drunk. Oh, it was early in the morning, and she had probably been limping around, feeling bad, and so they got out the little pint bottle of whiskey that everybody kept for medicinal purposes. Occasionally, when adults had a terrible cold, they'd have a hot toddy. I don't know what else went in it, but I know it had some of that whiskey.

And my mother was a snuff dipper. She had one of those little tin snuffboxes, not very big. She would buy a larger glass of snuff, which was sold in about an eight-ounce size with a seal over a tin top. She would scoop the snuff into her little tin box, and afterward we used the snuff glasses to drink out of. She also carried another little tin container to spit in. That snuff dipping is how my mother got cancer of the jaw. For dipping, she used a stick from a tree that grows all over the South. It had red berries and made a good toothbrush. We'd break off a section and chew the end of it to form the brush. She would do her teeth with a stick like that, but she'd also use one as a snuff dip. She'd twirl it around in that can and put it in her mouth. I used to have a big brown birthmark, and everybody said she had marked me because she took up snuff when she was pregnant with me. That mark faded away with age, thank God.

My sister and I tried that snuff one time, and we got so deathly sick. A big tree grew nearby the henhouse and draped a branch down over the roof. My sister and I would climb up and sit on the tin roof and smoke. We didn't think our mother could see us behind the branch, but she probably could if she looked out the window. When we thought we were hidden, we'd take rolling papers and put things in them. We tried this with grape leaves, and we smoked corn silk. One time we took some snuff and dipped it with little sticks. I got sick, but it made Ruth really sick; she was so sick that I told my mother what we had done.

I remember my mother working in the kitchen at the Methodist church once a week or maybe twice a month. We'd fix dinner for the Chamber of Commerce, and that's how we made money to furnish our parish and the pastor's home. Except for that, I don't remember my mother out in the community. Of course, people loved my mother; she had company all the time, and they felt comfortable in our home.

If you asked my mother, "How are you?" she made you think, "Sorry I asked you that" because she'd tell you how she was doing. She had varicose veins in one leg and would always say she'd had a "dark brown" or "light brown" headache. My older sister was exactly like her, just always sick with something. But my younger sister and I began to feel like sickness is next to nastiness, so I try not to ever complain, not to ever be sick. I always feel like it's about half nasty to be sick.

Our older sister was born sickly; very young, she had tachycardia. It's not life threatening; it's just one of those things. I take medication for it, too, a pill to keep my heart regulated. But Maggie was the first one to have it, and it manifested early, so my mother was very protective of her. Maggie picked up on that, boy, and never did a lick of work that she didn't have to; she dumped her work on me and Ruth. Ruth was a young beauty. Maggie and I looked alike—big nose and all—and we weren't that pretty. It didn't give us a complex or anything; we just knew Ruth was the pretty one. She looked different, like my grandmother. My mother put Ruth's hair up to keep her looking beautiful.

I guess I was a very curious child. I worked in the garden and in the yard all the time. I traded my sisters cooking and housekeeping and did outside chores because I liked being out. I started learning how to milk a cow when I was about five, and when I was about six, I had to milk my own cow every night and every morning. Then it increased to more—two cows, maybe. So every day we had a certain number of cows to milk in the morning before we went to school and at night when we got home. We'd put milk in a cream separator, either an old tin one or another one with a little window where you could see in. After the milk sat overnight, you'd let it out of the spigot and give that milk to the pigs. We drank whole milk, and we kept some of the cream. Once a week, somebody came by and picked up the cream. When we went to town, we'd take it to the creamery, where it was made into butter.

When we were kids, we were always hungry. We'd hunt for huckleberries and persimmons after the frost. We looked for passion vines, though that's not what we called them; they grew on the fence posts. Old pawpaws grew everywhere, and blackberries and dewberries crawled along ditches on the roads. Muscadine vines grew wild, but you don't find those anymore. Then there were possum grapes—we'd even eat those old possum grapes.

After school, we got off the bus at my grandmother Flanagan's house. She'd greet us, and we'd go with her through the house. She'd reach up in the cabinet and give us a biscuit with some bacon or a piece of cornbread with meat in it. Then she'd walk through her garden and part of the lane on our way home, and I can remember her pulling up green onions, stripping them down, and flipping the outer part off. We'd take off across the cattle lot and down the little path that led to our house a quarter mile away. I still think of how good that food was. Whether it was a cold biscuit or a slice of cornbread, she always had something for us.

My grandfather had a small cellar where he kept barrels of apples. He'd save apples from his orchard and wrap them in some kind of paper. The cellar always smelled like apples, and it was a big treat to go there when he made apple cider. He had a press of some kind, and we would turn and turn that thing, making cider.

We called our grandparents Mama and Papa Flanagan and spent a lot of time at their house. I used to work in the fields with Papa Flanagan, and I was the best pea picker of all his grandchildren. They had a whole bunch of us, for two other families with my first cousins lived nearby. But I was always the one who worked with Papa because I could keep up with him picking peas.

My grandfather was a tall, skinny man. He would squat instead of sitting in a chair. My dad asked him once, "Papa, do you ever think about dying?" Papa Flanagan said, "Foot, no. All I think about is living." In the South, they say "foot" instead of the other "F" word. He never cursed in front of us, although I think he did—I know he did—when we were not around.

In the summertime, I'd carry a jar of water down to him when he was working in the field between our houses if he was doing something I wasn't helping with. And a lot of the times, he'd give me a penny. Then I'd be there for a while, and he'd tell me about how he was going to buy me a horse.

He'd tell me all these tales—scary tales. I'd be sitting on his lap, and he would tell stories about panthers. We had panthers and even bears in our area of western Arkansas when I was growing up. They'd come around to eat once in a while, and he'd tell us how, when he was a young boy, the bears would come into their cabins occasionally. And he'd tell how, out hunting at night, they'd hear the scream of the panthers. We did, too; we didn't have many panthers in that area, but a few were still around. Oh, we'd be so scared!

My dad was deathly afraid of storms, especially tornadoes. My grandparents had a storm cellar dug in the side of the hill, and some nights they could tell we were going to have stormy weather. When it got bad, my dad would take us down there. I guess it was a fourth of a mile away, and we went stumbling down there with a little lantern in the middle of the night a few times. The storm cellar was just kind of a mound and had a door you'd open and go in. I couldn't have been more than about five years old, and it was deep enough for me to stand up in. But it was very little, very cramped, and it was kind of muddy on the bottom. As they moved the benches on the side to make room for us, they dug into the dirt on the side. Later, we built a concrete root cellar attached to the side of our house and used it as a storm cellar. And we put an extra room on top of it, with a covered breezeway into the kitchen. Mother put all of her canned goods and potatoes in there. It was a great relief for us because we had one of those spring beds in the new storm cellar so they could put us to bed. But when we were in the old storm cellar, my grandfather would tell ghost stories and scare us half to death.

My grandparents owned about a thousand acres. If you pictured our families' houses as forming a V, we lived at the point of the V, and my grandparents lived at the end of the left leg. My uncle and his family lived at the end of the right leg. Once a month, our cousins and all of us would meet at my grandparents' house; everybody brought something for a big noon meal. We spent a lot of time there, including for family reunions, until I went off to college.

My cousin Bequita lived in Paris, Arkansas, about thirty miles away; her dad was a postal worker. Once a month, we'd meet at my grandmother's for a big meal. At Christmas, my grandmother would clean out a cast-iron wash pot to cook the Christmas ham. Bequita's dad supervised the ham because he loved it. He'd pull the skin back after it was cooked and slice it up. We'd have vegetables from the canning, fried chicken, and all kinds of pie. My grandmother specialized in chess pie, which is like a custard pie.

They'd go out and get a Christmas tree for the Methodist church. It was always big, like the national Christmas tree, and one day we'd all go to the church and decorate it. We had a Christmas pageant at church that everybody attended. We would do plays, and I remember one time playing the role of Raggedy Ann, bending over like I was a rag doll. We also did readings, such as poems, and then we celebrated Christmas. Somebody would come all dressed up in a Santa suit and take gifts off the big tree. That is when everyone got their gifts because we didn't have a Christmas tree at home. We usually just got one or two presents, but we did have stockings at home. The greatest thing about my stocking was getting English walnuts, maybe two or three, and a big, fresh orange—yum—and an apple. Along with food in our stockings, we'd get maybe a pair of socks or something else that we needed and maybe little gifts.

Religion meant community to me as a child because the whole Grand Prairie community met at that Methodist church. We were a church. A circuit-rider minister from Charleston served the churches in Grand Prairie, Vesta, and one other town—three little satellite churches. He came one Sunday a month, and the rest of the time we had laypeople as speakers. We had Sunday school first, and then he did the service, probably after doing an earlier service and driving out.

We had a revival one time. I was just getting old enough to remember some of the preacher's sermons. When he told Bible stories, he would illustrate some of them dramatically. I have this image: he had a handkerchief, and he folded it up and cradled it, saying Delilah treated Samson like he was a little bitty baby.

Then the minister formed what he called booster clubs. He had one in Charleston and one in Grand Prairie, where he taught the kids a little song that went, "I'm a member of the booster club, the booster club." Anyway, he would have little lessons or fun songs to teach us social things basically.

Attending church was the big focal point of our weekend, and afterward we'd either go home with some of our friends, or they'd come home with us and spend the day. Then we'd go back to church Sunday night, and they'd go home with their families. About once or twice a year, the preacher would come home with us for Sunday dinner, stay all afternoon, and go back that night. The Methodist church was the only one in that community. It burned not too many years ago, but it had kept going for a long time and then merged with the Charleston church.

One of my great uncles was the superintendent of our Sunday school. Many Methodists had moved to the community, and most of them were also related to him. This great uncle had a deep scar down the side of his face, and he was black Irish. He had black hair and white skin that became brown from farmwork, which made the scar show even more. He was pretty strict with the kids and wouldn't let us make too much racket. If we were up to something, he would get after us, and sometimes I fantasized that he really was the devil. We went to their house on Sunday lots of times because they had a daughter the same age as my younger sister and a son my age, and we enjoyed riding their horses.

Saturday nights, we'd come into town from the farm to do grocery shopping and sometimes to go to a movie. We'd sit outside and watch the movie on a screen; the drive-in theater was there even when I was a young girl. We'd also go to the high school plays. That was a big deal—like going to the theater in New York, you know, to go to the high school play. I think the first movie I ever saw was *Red the Rose*. It was about the Civil War, I guess, and it was a big deal.

My dad took us to the Barnum and Bailey Circus one time. He had a ton-and-a-half flatbed truck, and he put bales of hay around the edges because the bed didn't have sideboards on it. He announced it ahead at Sunday school that he would take kids to town, and he took about twelve or fourteen kids who could afford the tickets. He drove us into Fort Smith to the Barnum and Bailey Circus—now that was a big deal. Dad was always kind of innovative; he'd do things like that for the whole community.

A traveling theater group, part of the old Chautauqua circuit, would come around and put on plays in tents. We'd drive into Charleston, about ten miles away, to see these little one-act plays. We'd also go to Branch, which was closer. That's where my mother's parents [her father and his second wife], Papa Callan and Mama, lived. I remember going over there and spending the night in a rattling old house. When they were younger, they had lived with her half-brother, his wife, and their three children, who were our contemporaries. We'd go over there once a month, at least, and spend the night, and I just remember these creaky ceilings and boards. They had an old clock that struck every half hour and every hour, and it would keep me awake. Every time that clock would strike, it would wake me up: boooonng. And then Papa, who was a hypochondriac, sat in the rocking chair, and his wife soothed him and took care of him, pampered him. He always drank goat milk, and he had to burp. He'd go, "Urrrrrr," long, drawn-out burps. It was the noise of those burps and of that clock that kept me awake.

Papa Callan had great big hands, but if we did something bad—if we'd stumble across his feet, be too noisy, or do something we weren't supposed to do around the dinner table—he'd thump us with those big old fingers. But it was wonderful to go there because they were sweet and wonderful, too. And I loved to go with my grandmother every night to milk the goat. She had hay stacked up, and the goat would put its front legs on this bale of hay and reach up to its tray of food on the top. Then the bag would hang out, and Mama would milk her. I helped her, and we had to drink the milk. We thought it was awful, but it probably didn't have any different taste.

Papa had an extensive orchard, and one of our chores was to take ashes from the fireplace and spread them around the fruit trees to keep the borers away. I still take out our fireplace ashes and put them around some of my trees because it's good for them. But I have really happy, wonderful memories of all my grandparents.

And I only had one spanking; no, I didn't even get a spanking, just a scolding. My girlfriend and I were playing cowboys with our milk cows out in the cornfield. After the harvest was over, we'd turn the cows out to eat the last of the corn and the stalks. We'd trained a couple of the cows to ride, and we'd taken cornstalks and were whipping the cows with them. My younger sister and I always had to get the cows out of the lower pasture when it was time to change pastures. And at night at the end of our chores, it was our job to go get the cows and bring them in. So instead of doing all that walking, which was probably a quarter mile away, we each had a cow we would ride. The Sunday we got in trouble, my girlfriend Irene King got on one of our cows and rode her. Irene whipped it with those cornstalks, playing cowboys and rodeo. Dad caught us, and, oh, did he get after us.

We got in trouble another time. When the oats or hay that we fed to the animals was ready, the threshing machine would come, with the neighbors taking turns getting their fields threshed. My mother would feed the workers, fixing big meals for everyone, when the threshing machine came to our house. One time, when I was between nine and twelve, the threshers had been there and had made a big pile of straw to feed the animals when it got cold. Sometimes in the winter, the animals would take shelter in the haystack, sort of dig into the side to stay warm.

It was a Sunday after church, and Ruth and Irene and I climbed to the top of the haystack. My dad was so angry; you don't ever disturb the hay until it rains because the rain settles it and packs down a kind of thatch that preserves the straw. You can't walk on the stacks because you make holes in them; then the rainwater gets down the holes, and the hay won't last as long. But we'd crawled up to the top of that haystack, and my dad came out yelling at us after we had walked around it about three times and made big holes in it. He hadn't told us not to do that, but I got a good, stern lecture. He tried to repair the holes we'd made, but I don't know how well that worked. I wasn't the leader, either; we were all doing it.

Then once we went swimming in the hog pond, which was probably deep in mud and not much water; I still remember the smell. Dad caught us and sent us down to another pond that was a lot deeper and clearer. We'd fished in that fresh pond some, but we were never allowed to swim in it because it was too deep; he had barred us from going in a couple of deep ponds. We thought he was going to give us and our cousins a spanking for swimming in that hog pond, just dog-paddling around. We were dripping wet, muddy, and cold, but he sent us to the other pond and came with us to be sure we could swim well enough to be in there.

I was looking through some pictures of Dale's forebears and mine, for our families are intermarried. My grandmother had seven children in her family, and my grandfather's family also had six or seven. Over the years, they were all married within that community. We were the fifth marriage between the four families, and we joke that it's almost incestuous but not quite. When I was speaking at a banquet in Bradford a few years ago, I realized how many relatives I still had down there. I was just astounded by how many first, second, and third cousins showed up and came up to talk. We grew up in the bosom of family in a great community—it was a good way to grow up.

CONNECTIONS

FAMILY AND FRIENDSHIP THROUGH THE YEARS[3]

BEQUITA BUMPERS GRAY[4]

In Little Rock, 2008, cousins Bequita and Betty talked about family history. Bequita recalls, "The Bumpers were French Huguenots among the first to flee religious persecution. There's only one family of Bumpers in the U.S., although there are some different spellings of the name. I think they originally came into Pennsylvania. Betty's mother was also of French Huguenot descent, and her full name was Ola Chastain Callan.

"The Callans and the Flanagans were Scotch Irish. Each of those families came up from Alabama in covered wagons to Arkansas. I think that's strange that they both came up from Alabama that way."

Bequita reflects on Betty's leadership, "The best thing about Betty is that she's always herself. She has a great way of surrounding herself with gifted people. She doesn't care much about detail, but she's good with vision. She attracts gifted people to help her.

"In the early days, Betty and I knew each other when they lived on the farm. Betty's father and my mother, Floy Flanagan, were brother and sister. I tell Betty that she is more like my mother than I am. I sing in the choir at church now, and when I look out at the congregation and see Betty, some of her gestures are so much like my mother. Brooke is more like me. Then, too, my daddy and Dale's daddy were brothers, so I am first cousin to Betty and Dale both.

"We used to tease Betty and Dale when they were dating that they were almost too related to each other, but not really. Betty and I have always been like sisters. She had two sisters and I had one, and we all went around together. Betty and I were especially close because she dated and married Dale.

"Betty and I were roommates at the University of Arkansas [Fayetteville]. That year Dale's parents were killed in a car crash. My family and I were from Vian, Oklahoma. Just before they were killed, Dale's mother and dad had been out to see my mother and dad in Vian. His parents were traveling with a married couple who were their neighbors. The husband, Harmon Flanagan, was the brother of Betty's dad and my mother. He was killed outright when a drunk driver hit their car. Within a short time, Dale's parents also died from their injuries.

"Betty and Dale had been engaged, and then they decided to get married that summer after his parents died. Dale was in law school, so when he finished, they came back to Arkansas. He was starting to practice law, and he worked in the store he had inherited from his dad. It was a furniture and hardware store, and my husband was in the same business, so we did a lot together. We were still in Vian, just to the west of Fort

Smith, and Charleston was just twenty miles away to the east of Fort Smith. We went to the markets in Fort Smith and shopped together. After his parents died, my mother and daddy were like parents to Dale.

Betty and Dale were a wonderful help to me the year I lost my family. My house burned, and it killed my husband and two children. My mother always believed that Dale was elected to save me. I came to Little Rock, and it gave me a new life and saved my sanity. I had always been a housewife, and I had mostly lived in Vian. In Little Rock, I started going around with Betty and her sisters and family, working on Dale's 1970 campaign. We traveled all around the state, campaigning. When he was elected governor, I worked as Dale's receptionist. I believe that a door never closes but another opens.

"Then in 1974, Dale was elected to the U.S. Senate, and they left to go to Washington, D.C. Just before that, when I was Dale's receptionist, a boy I had dated in high school came back to Arkansas. He'd been a friend of Dale's in high school. We had known each other a long time, he knew my family, and I knew his family, so we went out. I didn't think I would ever remarry, but we married. So I didn't go to Washington to work for Dale. Dale stayed with us when he was first in the Senate and came here to visit. Later, Betty and Dale rented an apartment here, then they bought a condo, and now they have a house here.

"Since the beginning of this summer [2010], Betty and Dale have been living in Little Rock. Betty is so adaptable, moving to Arkansas. It's a comfort to me that they are back. Betty and I are close, although we are different. She likes to do causes, and she doesn't really enjoy social things. I like to play bridge, entertain, and work in my church, and Betty likes to have a mission. She still does her immunization work with Every Child By Two.

"Their new house is great for them. It's not too big and not too little, and there's a garden in the back because Betty loves to garden. Their house is all on one level, and it is close to Brooke and her children. Brent's here, too, and Betty and Dale are the only people I know who are our age with such young grandchildren. Brooke's youngest is only seven, and Brent has one who's thirteen, so they were pretty old when the kids came. But Betty and Dale love it. I told them it was nice that their house was so close to Brooke, but they are too far from me. Betty just said, 'It's eleven minutes away.'

"This August we had a big birthday party for Dale. I think Dale is getting more relaxed, which is hard to do after you retire when you have always been so active. He still worked in Washington until they moved back here. The birthday party was called 'The Early True Believers' party, and it was for the people who first supported Dale when he ran for governor. It was such a clever idea. A lot of people who were the early supporters came from Charleston and Fort Smith, and Bill Clinton came.

It was a wonderful birthday party. Betty and Dale have created a great Arkansas legacy."

EXCERPTS FROM *THE BEST LAWYER IN A ONE-LAWYER TOWN*

DALE BUMPERS

In several passages of his memoir, Dale Bumpers recalls the struggles of the Flanagan family during the Great Depression:

> The H. E. "Babe" Flanagan family had moved to Ft. Smith from their upland farm, north of Charleston, in 1936. The plight of the family had been terrible, but things were beginning to look slightly better. Babe had three daughters and Betty was the middle one. Even though we had attended the same grade school, she was a grade ahead of me and we hadn't known each other.[5]

The following passage places the Flanagans' story in the broader context of economic conditions in northwestern Arkansas:

> They avoided starvation by growing enough food in the summer to carry them through the winter. Babe was a genius at trading anything for something else and coming out a little ahead. Two enviable qualities coalesced to save him and his family—determination and a creative mind. He conceived the idea of butchering a hog, grinding the whole carcass into sausage, and then hurrying off to Paris, a nearby community, with wife and children in tow, where they all went door-to-door peddling it. He netted five dollars on his first trip. This was more than all but a very few people were making per day.[6]

NOTES

1. Betty Bumpers, "Remarks," 2005 Induction, National Women's Hall of Fame, Seneca Falls, New York, Peace Links Records Addendum (unprocessed), Special Collections, University of Arkansas Libraries, Fayetteville.
2. "Franklin County," http://encyclopediaofarkansas.net/encyclopedia/entrydetail.aspx?entryID=410 (accessed July 15, 2012). Arkansas was a Confederate state during the Civil War. Confederate and Union bands engaged in Franklin County.
3. Anna Eblen's field notes, October 5, 2008, and phone conversations with Bequita Bumpers Gray, February 5, 2010, and August 16, 2010.
4. Bequita Bumpers Gray is a double first cousin to Betty and Dale Bumpers, and she is a lifelong friend. Bequita, called Quita, was Betty's childhood companion and then her college roommate. Bequita campaigned for Dale with Betty and other women from their families, and later she worked as a receptionist in Dale's office when he was Arkansas governor.
5. Dale Bumpers, *The Best Lawyer in a One-Lawyer Town* (Fayetteville: University of Arkansas Press, 2004), 54.
6. Bumpers, *The Best Lawyer in a One-Lawyer Town*, 72.

FIVE

Community on the Eve of World War II

We moved to Fort Smith from the farm when I was twelve. When I was a senior in high school, my dad decided to move the family back to Charleston—not back on the farm but to town. Both of those moves were turning points for me.

CONVERSATIONS WITH BETTY

When we moved to Fort Smith, here I was, this country girl who moved to town and a big junior high school. It was a whole new situation to cope with, and I learned a lot. One reason we moved there was that my dad had started trading and selling at a sale barn at Fort Smith. This was during the Depression, and there was no money in farming. My dad didn't particularly like farming, but he liked selling. As he established himself with this sale barn, he'd go back and forth.

Even though he was making some money, his absence was a burden on my mother. It was rough for her to have four children and to be left with all the chores: housework, milking, and taking care of the hogs that we had for winter meat. Back in those days in Arkansas, it was pretty depressing. She was burdened trying to do all of this work. Managing four kids—four kids who couldn't offer the same kind of help to her that he did—was too much.

She finally told him, "You know, it's either be home more to help with this work or get me off this farm. Or raise these children yourself—I'm not going live to raise these children."

So he just packed us up and moved us to Fort Smith, right in the neighborhood of that sale barn. And he was busy there: He'd buy a cow, maybe in the morning or whenever the sales rings first opened, and he might run her back in later on that afternoon to make five or ten dollars. Sometimes he would put a cow in his pickup truck and keep her a while in a pasture near our house and then sell her.

But he also kept the farm near Charleston, and sometimes he'd take cows there to fatten them up or breed them or put them out to pasture, depending on the time of the year, and then bring them back to Fort Smith. If a cow was already bred and bumping a calf, he'd take it home until closer to birthing. He'd wait until the cow had her calf and then take them both back to the auction barn and sell them. And he made money that way.

I don't remember what all we did to help out, but my mother made us iron laundry and cook one meal a day. When we were growing up, we kept dust rags in a drawer at every entrance to our house because the minute our dad came in and caught us lolling around on the couch or something, he'd call us trifling. We'd jump up and grab a skirt and a dust rag—the skirt because we had these little shorts outfits with skirts that matched, and he didn't like us wearing just the shorts. And we'd grab the dust rags to keep from being called trifling.

We had a milk cow at that time, and that was my job, too; I mowed and milked. I didn't like cooking or cleaning house, but my two sisters liked inside work better than outside. At Fort Smith, I remember going seven blocks to the pasture where we kept our milk cow. My dad rented the pasture, and he would also keep cows there that he bought short term instead of taking them back to the farm, nearly thirty miles away. I would go there every morning and afternoon to milk the cow and bring the milk home. I did that for two or three years, and then we moved to a larger place on the edge of town that had a bigger pasture.

I remember one incident from when we first moved to Fort Smith very well because I had just had my hair cut at the barber. I liked the idea of being a boy, so I had a boy haircut. It was parted and brushed back, a little Dutch girl thing, but it was a boy haircut. Both of my sisters had bangs and short bobs.

The first day I went to junior high in Fort Smith, I was in the second half of the seventh grade. It was the only junior high school for the second-largest city in Arkansas, so it was a big school. We went into this castle-looking building, a four-story junior high school that had these old-style turrets. They had a room I will never forget. It was room 318, and it was in a turret. But you had to go through room 319 or 317 to get to that room, and I couldn't find 318. There was no sign, or I missed the signs, and I ended up running from the fourth floor down to the next floor, all through the halls and to the basement, about three times. I remember just panicking. I was frantic for those five minutes between classes, trying to find that classroom. And I finally ended up in despair, standing against a locker—somewhere around 318, I guess—sobbing because I was so exhausted. Finally a teacher came by and said, "What is wrong?" And I said, "I can't find room 318." The teacher led me in there, and I was so embarrassed. I had a snotty nose, and I was crying. Anyway, that was a traumatic experience, but I realized that what you need to do is ask someone. Don't panic; ask!

When you move into a community like that or into a situation like that, it's true what they say—that birds of a feather flock together. I was different, and my closest friends were young women from a Catholic orphanage. I mean, we were kind of marginalized. They seemed that way to me, and I was, too. Here I was—this girl with a haircut like a boy's and homemade dresses. I was clean (but different looking) and new, coming in at the middle of the year. And so these girls became some of my earliest and best friends. I've kept up with seven of them for a long period of years, and they all turned out to have successful lives. Later on, I made other friends, too, and adjusted and had a great life in Fort Smith.

When we first arrived, we heard President Roosevelt's inauguration speech broadcast over the loudspeaker in a huge assembly. The seventh, eighth, and ninth grades were sitting in the auditorium and listening when he said, "The only thing we have to fear is fear itself." We all got to convene and hear the radio, which was thrilling because radios were relatively new and not many people had them. Of course, I had heard my dad talk about Roosevelt. We were all taught, jokingly, that when we died, instead of going to God, we were going to Franklin Roosevelt. Roosevelt brought electricity to our farms, and he brought city sewers and water to Charleston. Actually, when Roosevelt came in, it was the first time the South had not been treated as a conquered nation. And that's why I have always had such great respect for his work.

In my teen years, I had a horse. Oh, I was so in love with my horse that I didn't discover boys until later. We kept my horse on a pasture for the four years that we lived in Fort Smith. We liked to take long rides, off far away. I fell in love with that horse when I was twelve, and I was still in love with it, but when I was sixteen or seventeen, I discovered boys. I started dating in the tenth grade and had a boy I liked quite a lot.

I was sometimes very competitive, more so than most people. I wanted to win. I was not active in team sports because we were in high school during World War II, when schools were bare bones. All the guys were gone, and we had no coaches, no male teachers, no football team. I missed a lot, not being able to play basketball or some competitive sport in high school.

Another turning point in my life was moving back to Charleston because we moved in the summer before my senior year in high school. I had all these friends—including a sweet romance. That first dating experience was with a boy I liked a lot, and it was hard having to move off. I never questioned my family; I just accepted the fact that we were moving to Charleston and too bad if I wanted to stay up there in high school. I don't remember even protesting, even saying, "I don't want to move my senior year. I want to go to school here. I want to stay in school in Fort Smith." I mean it just wasn't a choice. I did stay there for several days with a friend because I was teaching at vacation church school. I taught young, young kids and couldn't leave until I had finished that.

My dad decided to move us back to Charleston because he'd started trading cattle and had this idea about Jersey cows. He was a real trader, and he made enough money that we stayed in town and didn't go back to the farm. That was the summer I met Dale and we started dating. Though we had cousins in common, we didn't really meet until high school. Our ages were six months apart, but he was a year behind me in school because of his August birthday. I had started school the year before due to my January birthday. At first I thought Dale was arrogant—he had a handkerchief collection, with a handkerchief from each girl he'd dated. He wanted mine, and I said no, and that was a challenge to him. I was already crazy about a boy in Fort Smith. In a little town like Charleston, Fort Smith was a big city, and Dale was jealous. My sister was dating Dale's brother, so we double-dated to the movies some, in the beginning.

I didn't have a lot to do with my classmates in Charleston because I was all enthralled with Dale. I didn't develop many close friends in my senior class because, having moved, I had not known most of them before. Maybe I'd known their families or a little bit about them because I had gone through the first seven grades with some of them when I was bused in from the country. I was much closer to my Fort Smith friends. I missed them a lot, and I'd go up there when I could to ball games. My Fort Smith boyfriend would meet me at the ballgames, and I'd stay with girlfriends.

When Dale and I were dating, I taught him to dance at my house, and he talks about this in his book *The Best Lawyer in a One-Lawyer Town*. Dancing reminds me of a true story about the Methodist minister and the Baptist preacher in Charleston. When the high school scheduled a senior prom that included dancing, the Baptist preacher was upset and approached the Methodist minister. The Baptist preacher said, "We should go down to the high school together to talk to the students about dancing." The Methodist minister said, "Brother Harding, I don't think they'd dance with us."

When we lived in Fort Smith, we went to a Methodist church, and I was active in the MYF (Methodist Youth Fellowship). That's where the young people's social life was. It was called the Epworth League when I first started attending. When we moved to Charleston, that's how Dale and I got the car for dates because his dad would let him have the car to pick me up for MYF. If Dale couldn't get the car, I got Dad's pickup truck. Dad had both a car and a truck, and I loved driving the pickup truck because that is how I had learned to drive. So I would sometimes get Dale and go to MYF. We would drive to Paris, Arkansas, real fast and get a

Coke. It was an adventure to ride down there. Being in the MYF was just part of my growing up.

My dad was kind of a visionary when he got the idea of transporting Jersey cows and selling them in Iowa. He introduced them there when the concept of dairies was beginning to form. Before, people would have a cow or two and sell milk in their own community, but as the population grew and people wanted pasteurized milk, large dairies started to develop. In the South, we had fine Jersey cows, and Dad sold these up north.

Jersey cows are little, compact, and their milk has very high butterfat content. They're beautiful, small cows with great big old eyes and dish faces. In Iowa and South Dakota, dairies had to keep them in barns because the snow was so deep during the terrible, cold winters up there. These little Jersey cows were easy to winter in a barn because they didn't eat a lot, and they gave this wonderful, rich milk—a lot of milk for a small cow. Milk was sold by the butterfat content then, and theirs was rich in butterfat.

My dad had become quite successful, and it was easier to operate out of the farm in Charleston. He had his own trucks, trailers, and tractor-trailers by then, and he'd buy truckloads of cattle. Even though my dad started out with trucks, he tried shipping cattle by rail. My brother would ride in the caboose and take care of the cattle when the trains stopped at certain places. I don't think that worked out too well because he didn't do that for very long.

They would buy and haul the cattle mostly by truck, and they attended private sales all over Iowa and South Dakota. That was where my dad started making a lot of money. My brother, who by this time was married, living on the farm, and managing it, would also go to cattle sales. My dad would drive back and forth, hauling cattle to Iowa, and he usually had a man, besides my brother, who went along in the truck.

In the summertime, sometimes he would send me, instead, with a loaded truck. We would stop at certain places to take care of the cows along the way. After so many hours, we'd have to let them out and give them water and food, and we'd milk some of them. Often a cow would be birthing a calf, and we'd help take care of that. When we reached Iowa, Nebraska, or South Dakota, we would unload them in barns and tend to them there, too. I remember going up to the Ozarks one time and being so bored. We were going so slowly up those mountain roads that I'd get out and walk.

I would work in a sale ring at the barns, demonstrating what fine milk cows we had. I'd squirt milk up to the top of the sale barn and try to hit somebody with it. Lots of trading was going on; my dad and my brother went to private sales each week, and those two would ham it up in the sale barns.

Sometimes, coming back, I remember putting up a hammock across the sideboards of the truck, getting in, and sleeping in there. The hammock would be under the roof of the front part of the truck, though I'd move it in hot weather. When we were hauling cattle, the hammock would hang just above the cows' heads. I didn't do too much traveling because we also were busy with the dairy we had on the farm. The three of us sisters were in charge of it, and I delivered milk.

That dairying went on until the laws changed so that milk was sold by bulk weight instead of butterfat content. Then my dad started hauling other loads with his trucks. Instead of bringing back an empty truck, he tried to make contacts and find someone who needed a load hauled back to Arkansas. Or he'd buy a truck full of grain, maybe, just to keep from driving an empty rig back. He started buying three-day-old calves because once a cow gives birth, it takes three days to get the colostrum out of her milk. You can't put colostrum into dairy milk, so that means keeping a cow out of production until at least three days after the calf is born. Farmers would keep the calves, let them suckle for three days, and then have no use for them.

My dad wanted only heifer calves, so he'd buy those. He'd pay a dollar a head—it's hard to imagine just a dollar a head for these three-day-old Jersey calves. And then I became an expert on how to keep a calf alive because those three-day-old calves would get scours—that's what we called diarrhea—and we'd feed them with a bucket of milk. We'd buy dozens and dozens of eggs because eggs would bind them up and give them nutrition. And, boy, I'd go up to a calf, open its mouth, crack an egg, and let that raw egg go down.

Later, my dad hooked up with an old man named Colonel Piper at one of the sales. He was a lot older than my dad and had been a racehorse auctioneer. He wore about six or eight diamond rings and was always dressed in a suit and a necktie. He was a pale, brown-eyed blond, although he was gray at that time. The Colonel was a fastidious man, even though he didn't take baths. He stayed with us a lot, and mother would always try to get him to take a bath. He wouldn't do that, as he thought it was unhealthy. He never had an odor about him, though, so he evidently used a washrag and washed himself up all the time.

Colonel Piper saw the potential in what my dad was doing, so he joined my father's business. Even though the Colonel was at the end of his career, he helped arrange sales. Colonel Piper was the auctioneer at these, but my dad would make little speeches, too. Colonel Piper stayed with the business for ten or fifteen years, until he died; he died in our home. My dad learned a lot from him, and they made a lot of money and bought a lot of farmland.

My dad was known all over Iowa and South Dakota for his cows and milk, and he stood by his cows. If a cow didn't turn out to be good or if it turned out to have only three teats, he usually gave people their money back. Or sometimes he would trade another cow. He was very honest, and people knew it, after he did that for several years because reputation travels fast in that community.

He made a lot of money at it, a lot of money. My dad died a wealthy man, not wealthy-wealthy but wealthy in that community. He continued to go back and forth on trips and was still trading cattle up to a few years before he died. They also traded in quarter horses, and I'd go along to demonstrate the horses, showing their gaits and what fine horses they were. I got bucked off several times. But neither of my sisters would show them because they didn't like horses. They didn't like any of that kind of traveling or selling and trading, but I did. I'd go along, and I learned a lot. When I was at Iowa State, Dad would come by to see us; if we had any break and the sale was very close to Ames, I'd go out and help him.

Just after I graduated from high school, my dad bought an ice cream parlor close to the high school at Fort Smith that sold sandwiches and had curb service. Two of our male cousins had been drafted, and their mother, a widow, was my mother's best friend. She was desperate to sell this ice cream shop, which they had owned and operated, so my dad bought it and put me and my sister Maggie, who was at Fort Smith Junior College, to work there. Ruth was still in high school, so for a year the two of us ran this ice cream shop and sold sandwiches to the kids at Fort Smith senior high school. We would have lunch and a malt or ice cream at the shop and then go to work. The shop was open at night, so we took an apartment at Fort Smith

In the summer before his senior year in high school, Dale came in while we were running the ice cream shop. His sister lived in Fort Smith, and he stayed with her and worked at Kroger's store during the summer. So we continued to date. This was during the height of World War II, 1942 to 1943, and we ran that shop pretty successfully. Then Maggie and I both decided that we wanted to go on with our education. So my parents sold the shop, and the new owners ran it successfully for several years because it was so close to the high school. It was a good thing, just not what we wanted.

When Maggie and I were in Fort Smith working at the ice cream shop and deciding to go on with our education, my dad was still traveling back and forth to Iowa selling cattle. A lot of my social life was with Dale that summer before his senior year. With his sister living in Fort Smith, he'd drive the twenty-three miles from Charleston and stay with her on weekends so we would see each other.

My dad decided to move the family to Iowa because Maggie had started dating a soldier, and we were almost forbidden to date soldiers in Fort Smith because he thought it was risky. But Fort Chaffee, an army base, was there, and everybody dated soldiers. I didn't because I still had a lot of high school friends that I ran around with, and I dated boys who were coming back.

Dale left to go to the University of Arkansas at Fayetteville in the summer of 1943 after he had graduated from high school. Dale's brother was already in the army, and he knew that he could be drafted at any time while he was at the university. Maggie was dating and had become quite serious with a soldier from Pennsylvania whom she later married. My younger sister was dating a boy in Charleston, a big football hero, but he was somebody my mother and dad didn't approve of. So dad thought, "I'll just kill two birds with one stone. I'll move my wife and three girls to Iowa State." So that's what he did. He bought a house in Ames and moved us lock, stock, and barrel, thinking that he would break up my sisters' romances. Of course, they both ended up marrying the men he was trying to get them away from. One of them, Ruth, later divorced, and the other one, Maggie, lived with her husband very happily forever, until they both died in their eighties. Later on Maggie's husband Archie kept the accounts for my father's trading business; he helped my dad make a lot of money over the years.

Before college, while Dale and I were dating, I was also dating the other Fort Smith boy I mentioned, and Dale had some other girlfriends. We didn't restrict dating; we dated other people. As it turned out, he went into the service, we went to different colleges, and we were doing all kinds of separate things. While he was in the service, he dated women at the different places he was stationed. When we were away from each other, we always wrote, and we always maintained this love for each other. With his being in the service for three years, we courted for about nine years.

When we moved to Ames, I ended up at Iowa State, and about that time Dale went into the armed services. He was drafted after he was in summer session at the university; he joined the Marine Corps and left for boot camp. I still have the trunk full of all the love letters that I got from Dale. While I was at Iowa State, I'd come home to Charleston when Dale got leave. My dad would, very thoughtfully, let me drive there with him, as he was going back and forth to ship cattle. My dad and my brother still were working at the farm and still buying Jersey cattle to send to Iowa. But my dad was living with us in Ames more than he was in Arkansas, as he went to sales all over Iowa, South Dakota, and Nebraska.

At Iowa State, I didn't know what I wanted to be or to do, so I started out majoring in landscape architecture. I loved gardens and farming, and I thought it would be great as a career. Then I took my first class and allowed myself to be intimidated out of it because I was the only girl. I sometimes wonder how in the world women could overcome that feeling, but they did. Even in the nineteenth century, some women overcame it, and even before that, a few overcame intimidation and succeeded as doctors and lawyers. When I started studying landscape architecture, the additional requirements filled up the first two years, and after I realized I was the only girl in the major, I changed to an art major.

I did not do well in college. It was a huge campus, and army, navy, and armed services training programs were going on. They were called things like V12, V8, V5, and they were all specialized; it was tough, exacting training that the servicemen went into. One big dorm was for training naval chefs and cooks. Though it was called a chef school, it really just taught the men to be cooks for the navy. We dated some of those servicemen, and I think the chef bit got added because the guys were hoping to be assigned as the chef on a ship. But mostly, they ended up just cooking for the naval barracks.

School was on the quarter system, and we started in September, with each quarter three months long. My older sister ended up leaving and getting married after one quarter. Then Ruth and I finished up the first year and started our second year, but we'd skip classes. Oh, God; I wasn't wild and wasn't drinking or anything at that age, but I think maybe we experimented with alcohol a little bit, not much. I did start smoking cigarettes when I was twenty-one. It got to be a craving because I found it relaxing. It was a tactile thing for me, something to do with my hands.

And, of course, we had many friends because we sisters were unusual: You didn't see many Southern girls on the Iowa State campus. We laughed all the time about being at a cow college. Of course I was very slim and trim in those days, and with being three sisters in school, we created quite a little splash, three Southern girls. I just played a lot those first two years—more than I should have. My younger sister Ruth, who was so pretty, was known as a beauty on campus. We pledged a sorority, and that took up a lot of time. It was all a different world to me, but it was not our cup of tea. We did have the girls from the sorority out to our house there in Ames, and they loved coming because my mother always liked company. As we'd grown up, my mother thought we could have all the company we wanted because my dad traveled all the time. She just wanted us at home so she knew where we were and what we were doing.

In Fort Smith, all the MYF kids had hung out at our house, and the same thing happened at Iowa State. The girls from the sorority would come and spend the weekends, and instead of studying, we just played and giggled and carried on. We lived in town the first year, and for the second year, I didn't want to move into the sorority house. I think you had to have a three-point grade average to be initiated and live there; I never ever hit that, so I was never initiated. But I was not that interested in the first place. We hadn't even known what sororities were until we moved to Ames and the woman next door got us interested in pledging. Though it didn't work out too well, it was fun, and we enjoyed the friendships and activities. I did stay in touch with a number of the girls for a long time, but the three I really stayed in touch with were the girls I shared a room with in the dorm.

When our friends came over, we just did what girls do. We would make each other up, or, if one of them were going on a date or out somewhere, we would dress them up. We'd go to movies or hang out together. We did maybe get all excited about dates because there weren't many boys around. The fellows who were on campus with government programs were kept so busy they had very little free time, although we all dated a few of them. But there was just no time left for them or for us between the studies and training.

While we were away in school at Iowa State, my grandmother Flanagan died. My parents went to her funeral, but none of us girls could go because our term was in session. My grandfather lived to be eighty-three, and he always lived in the same house in Grand Prairie near where I grew up. His oldest son lived there in my grandfather's old age and took care of him. Papa Flanagan would visit his other children, but he never stayed more than three days, at the longest, before he wanted to go home.

During my first year at Iowa State, Franklin Roosevelt died, and I remember how devastated we were. Of course, living on a dirt farm in rural Arkansas, we'd loved him. Everyone was all tense and upset about the war, and then Roosevelt died. I remember all of us sitting and listening to the news and the announcement. It was a tough, tough time.

Also that year, our cousins Bequita and Bernice came to visit us. They were Dale's and my mutual cousins, as their mother was a Flanagan, the sister of my father, and their father was the brother of Dale's father. We were just so busy with personal life, plus school, plus friends visiting, and my dad traveling back and forth—mostly we just had a fabulous time. In Arkansas, my brother Callans had married and had his first two babies, two sons only eleven months apart. At the end of that first year, my mother didn't want to stay in Ames. My dad wasn't there that much, Maggie had left, and I think mother had had it up to here with three girls and all of our sorority friends, college friends, and extended family friends. She was just exhausted from all of this taking care of girls. When my brother and his wife had the two babies, she wanted to move home, so dad moved her home.

Ruth and I went back to Iowa State and spent our second year living in a dorm. Though I had finished that second year at Iowa State, my younger sister, who, as I said, was a beauty, didn't do well in school. She dated a lot, and she flunked out of Iowa State when she did not maintain the required 2.5 grade average. She dropped out after the second quarter and got married. She was two years younger than I was, and she was just too young for college. She hadn't done her last two years of high school because she was very smart and a straight-A student. I was not; I was a B, C, and D student in high school because I was a daydreamer even then.

Looking back now, I realize that I suffered from a degree of narcolepsy. When I sit still very long, if I am not totally engaged in something, I just fall asleep easily. It happened at college lots of times, in the lecture halls. Of course, I also wasn't keeping good hours. I didn't sleep a lot, but I have always been a crazily erratic sleeper. My mother said my brother and I were her problem sleepers; she could never get us to bed at night, and then we would beat her out of bed every morning.

I did not go back to Iowa State for the third year because I had an appendectomy four days before I was supposed to leave for Iowa, and they kept me flat on my back for twelve days. Back in those days, they didn't let you get up. I developed an abscess in the incision and walked humped over for three weeks. You know, it was serious! It's a wonder I didn't die of peritonitis. Probably being a strong farm girl was the reason I didn't. My sister Ruth watched the operation. They let her stand in the operating room without a cap, or gown, or anything.

After I didn't return to Iowa State because of the appendectomy, I started teaching art in Charleston. I filled in for a teacher who was pregnant, as pregnant women were not allowed to teach back then. I filled out the rest of the full year, and I thought, "You know, I really like teaching; I like early childhood education." In the meantime, I was dating Dale while he was in the service. I also dated other friends who would come in and out of town, and I sort of fell in love with another fellow from Charleston, and we would go out when he was home on leave.

There were five girls—Ruth, Bernice, Bequita, Maggie, and me—without much to do on summer evenings when we were home. My sister Maggie's husband, Archie, was gone for three years in Europe, and the husband of one of the cousins was gone for three years. Ruth's husband, Lewis, had a 4F deferment and couldn't go in the service, so the two of them would go out with us. Lewis was a used car salesman, and he and Ruth lived in Fort Smith.

My dad recognized that we needed some outlet for our energy, so he would take us dancing. He and mother would take us to the Twenty One Club with whatever fellows were around. We all had friendships with high school kids from Fort Smith and Charleston, and we'd go out dancing. That was when I had my first drink, and that's how I know I wasn't drinking in college. My dad introduced us by letting us have mixed drinks with him. He'd get up and dance with all of us, and he was a wonderful dancer. He didn't know any of the dance steps, but we did all the jitterbugging. He was a good straight rhythm dancer, which I still prefer to anything else.

On weekends, we were entertained pretty royally, going with my dad to several different nightclubs in Fort Smith. I never could stand the thought of getting drunk because I wanted to be in control. I always wanted to know where I was and what I was doing, and I didn't ever have any desire to drink so much that you lose control of yourself and behave in a certain manner. But my older sister would occasionally drink too much. And I remember my dad laughing about it and just letting her do it once or twice. That kind of cured her, and she never drank much after that. That's how we passed the war years with nobody around. We didn't even have a football team my last year of high school in Charleston because there weren't enough fellows around.

But I still wanted to go to school, and this relates to my cousin. He had got out of the service, and even though his mother was a widow and they didn't have money, the GI Bill enabled him to go to school. I don't know how he found the Academy of Fine Arts in Chicago, but he went there and loved it. The school was really a design school; it offered dress and hat design. He talked me into going up there, so the next fall, I did.

In Chicago, I lived in the same building as my cousin. He had taken a room on the south side with a widow who had an extra bedroom. People were renting out rooms a lot because we didn't have the option of hotels and motels. The widow's building was very close to the YWCA, so he arranged for me to stay there at first. A doctor's family lived in the apartment above hers, and they only had one child. He was a podiatrist, and I guess he was having a hard time making a living. Both apartments had two bedrooms, and they agreed to rent me the bedroom like the one my cousin had downstairs. The room had a single bed that was their young daughter's. The wife didn't like to get up in the morning, so she agreed to rent the room if I would get up and fix her daughter's breakfast and get her off to school. It cut down some on my rent, so I did that. The daughter would go off early, and that was the end of my duties with her for the day.

My cousin and I would take the elevated train downtown to school. He had already been there one year, and in the middle of that year, he got a job offer from a milliner in The Fair Store. Marshall Field was considered the best department store in Chicago, and Carson Pirie Scott was the next biggest, with The Fair Store third. This woman hired him in the millinery department because, I think, he was already working for her part-time to supplement his GI Bill.

The Fair Store had a huge millinery department in the basement and then another, fancier one up on the second or third floor. He quit school to work with her, and I would go there after school and do some work for him because I was more creative and a better seamstress than he was. The store had fancy hats, and I remember designing some of them for him. We had these big frames and netting, and I'd twist that netting and put flowers and feathers in it. That was part of my schoolwork, too—designing—and I would design some of the most gorgeous hats. I'd go home and put them together. It was fun working for him, and we had a great time.

After work at the store, a lot of times my cousin and I would go to a bar and have a drink and then catch the elevated train home. My cousin always had all these cadres of friends—good-looking, handsome, young men—and I would just flirt my tail off with them, not realizing that they were gay. I mean, I could not understand it, and it sort of gave me a complex. They were so friendly and nice, and I knew they liked me; we would have such a good time. But they never, ever asked me out on a date. And, you know, I never did figure that out until after I left there and after he moved to another city when he got a fabulous job with another millinery company. Later, he became very wealthy through the business; when Dale was in law school, we used to go visit him. We were always close, and I continued to visit with him and his partner until my cousin died three years ago. But that year in Chicago brought that little encounter with a gay community that I didn't know anything about. All these good-looking boys, and they weren't the least bit interested in me.

That was an eventful year, when I did wonderful, exciting things. My cousin and I took advantage of whatever Chicago had to offer, as much as we could afford. There were lectures, and then, of course, the Art Institute was up the street from the Academy of Fine Arts on Michigan Avenue and had a lot of functions. I had to work pretty hard because we put on our own fashion show and had to design and do the patterns and buy the fabric. I had to have, I think, five costumes by the end of the year, including a beaded gown, so fashionable and proper, and a suit. School was tough, and I really had to work hard. I made some good friends there, too, whom I stayed in touch with for years.

At the end of that year, Dale came home to Charleston. That next summer, when I went home, my dad just did not like the idea of my going back to Chicago. I was pretty good; I could have gone on to work with designers or with some fashion house. A couple of fellows I knew were starting their own design business, and one of them became quite a famous dress designer on Seventh Avenue in New York. Later, he tried to get me to come to work for him; we stayed in touch even after Dale and I married. Anyway, my dad just said, "That is a tough business, Betty, and it is not something I think you ought to try to go into." He understood better than I did that I was not that committed to a career.

Dale was going back to the University of Arkansas, and I decided to go there the next year instead of to Chicago, and, of course, Dale and I dated. Dale decided to go to law school, and he met the requirements, which in those days were to have at least eighty-three hours and a B average. He was accepted at Northwestern University Law School, in Evanston, Illinois, after we had been at the University of Arkansas together and dating for a year.

My cousin Bequita also went to the University of Arkansas and became my roommate. Bequita and I had an apartment off campus, and that's when I really buckled down and studied and made pretty good grades. She was a good student, and I learned how to study through her. She had a dilemma, as did I, about whom to marry. In my junior year, in painting class, we were presented with a canvas and told to express ourselves. Nothing came to me. I have no inner drive to express myself, no vision inside. So I switched to studying to be an art teacher, and I was good at that. I'm not an artist, just a good mechanic. But I could help kids turn their work into something good—I showed them how to turn a squiggle into a frog. I decided to study teaching because I enjoyed it.

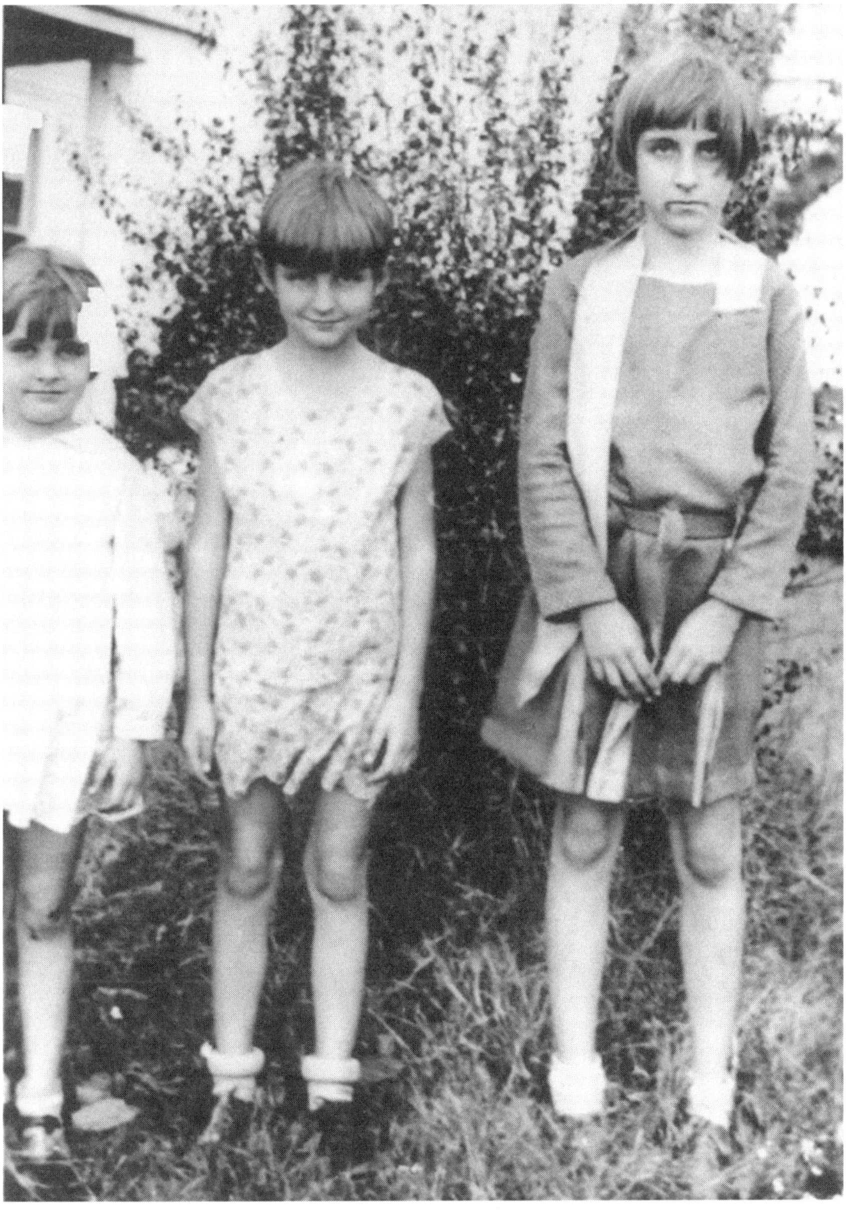

Sisters Ruth, Betty, and Maggie Flanagan as children

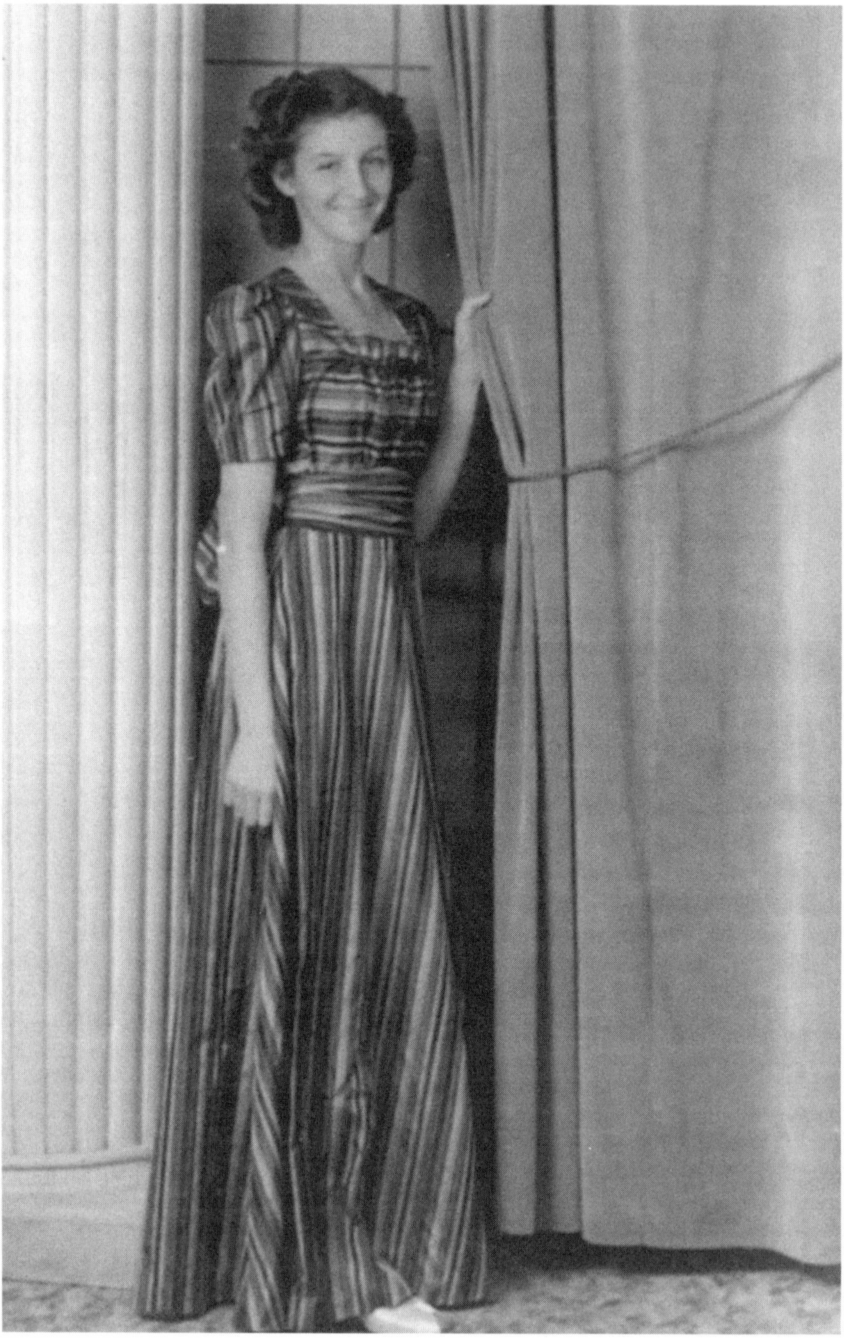

Betty Flanagan's first formal dress, sixteen years old

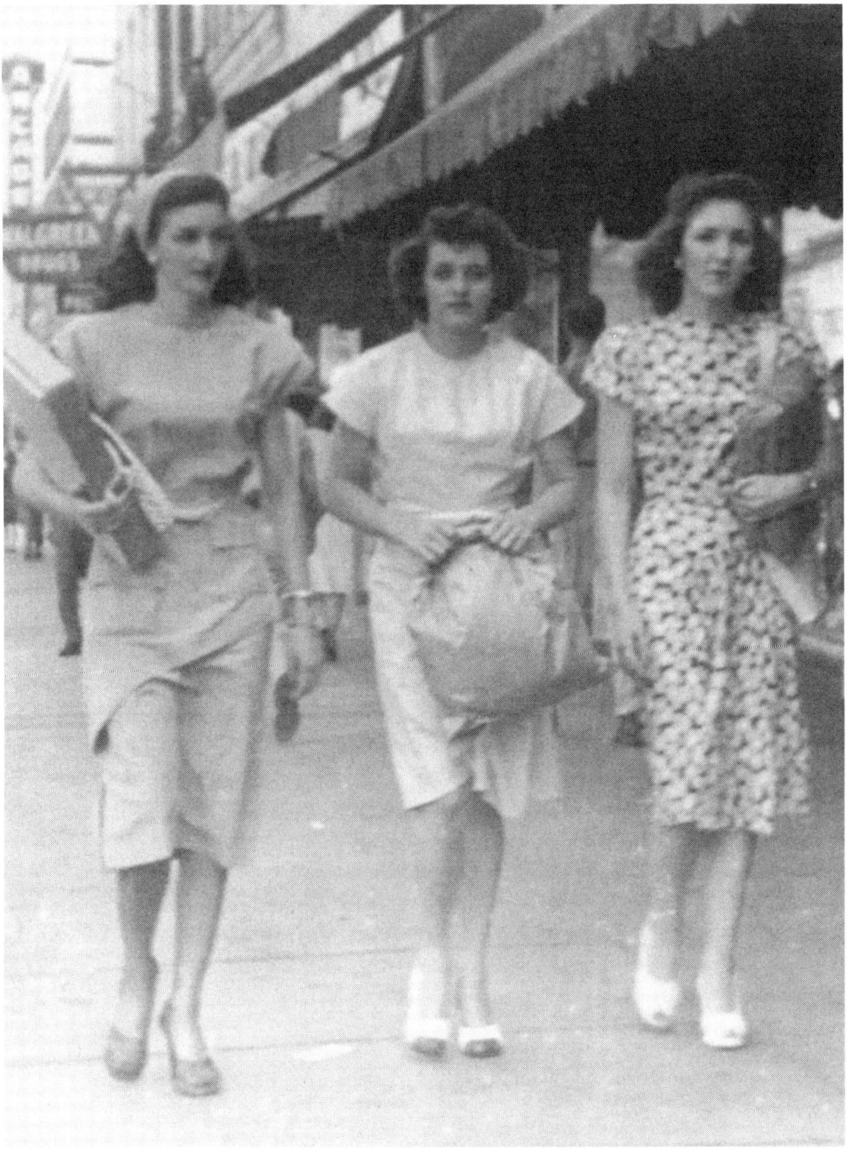

1948 street photo: Betty Flanagan, sister Ruth Wolfe, and cousin Bernice Bumpers Cary

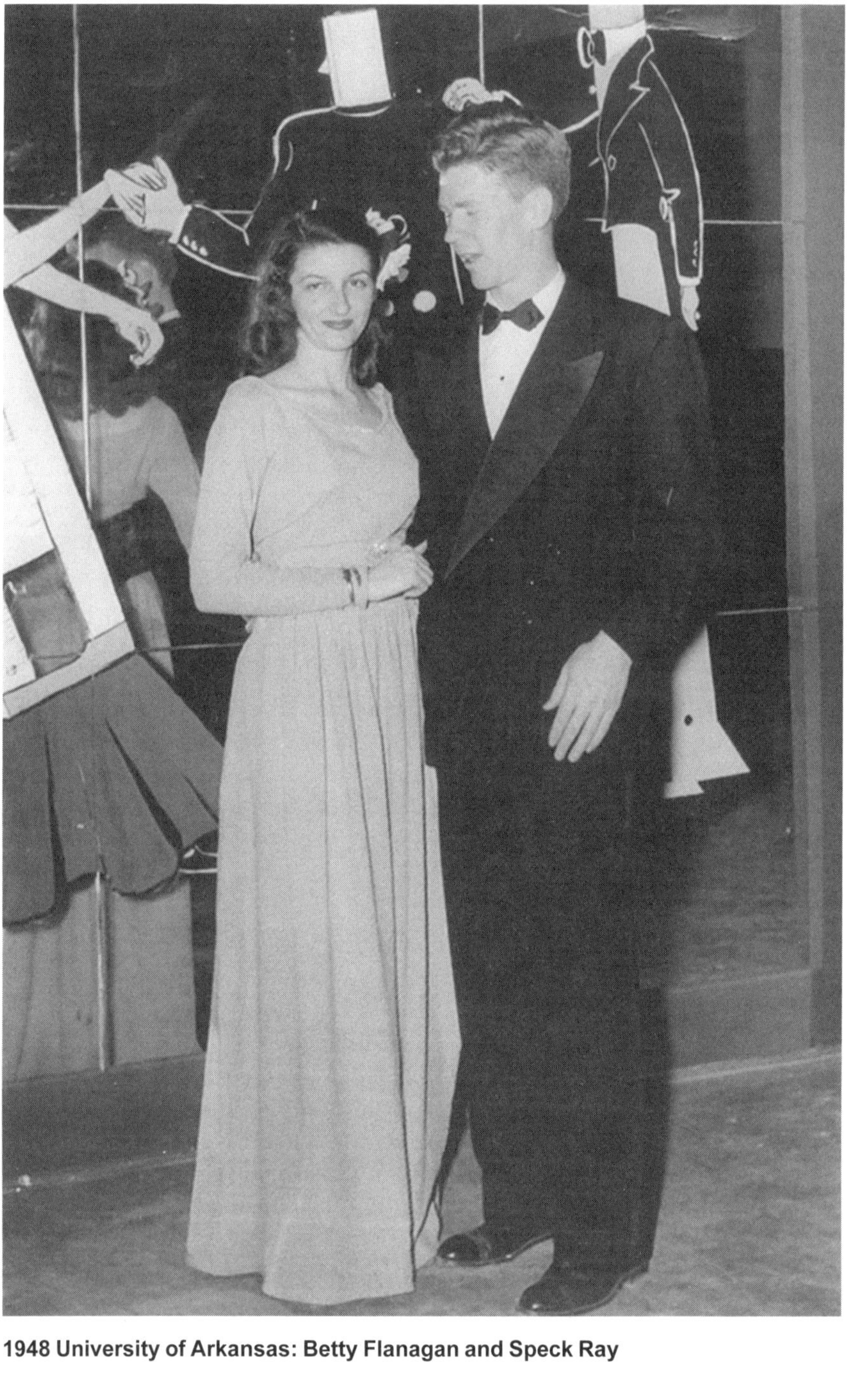

1948 University of Arkansas: Betty Flanagan and Speck Ray

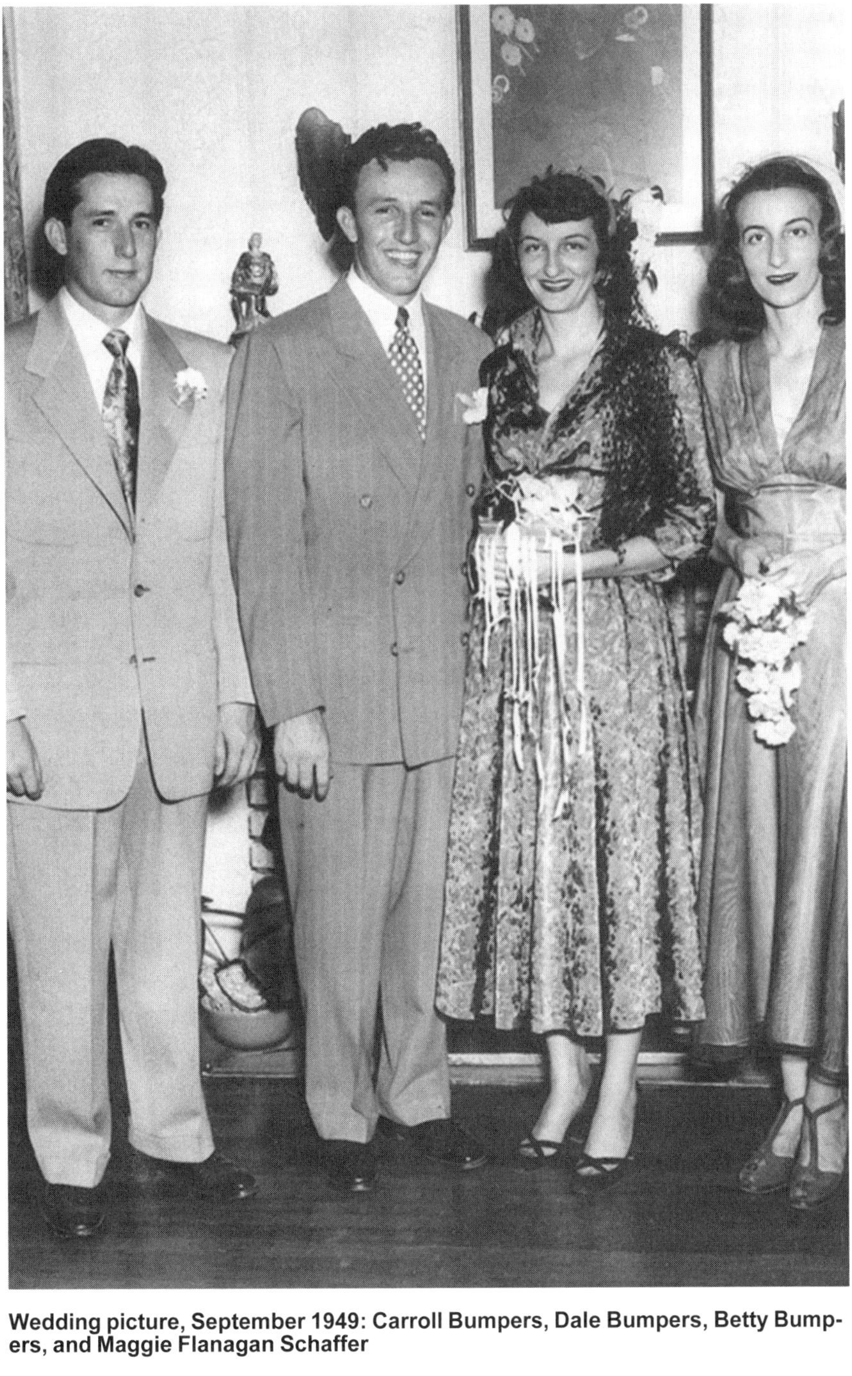

Wedding picture, September 1949: Carroll Bumpers, Dale Bumpers, Betty Bumpers, and Maggie Flanagan Schaffer

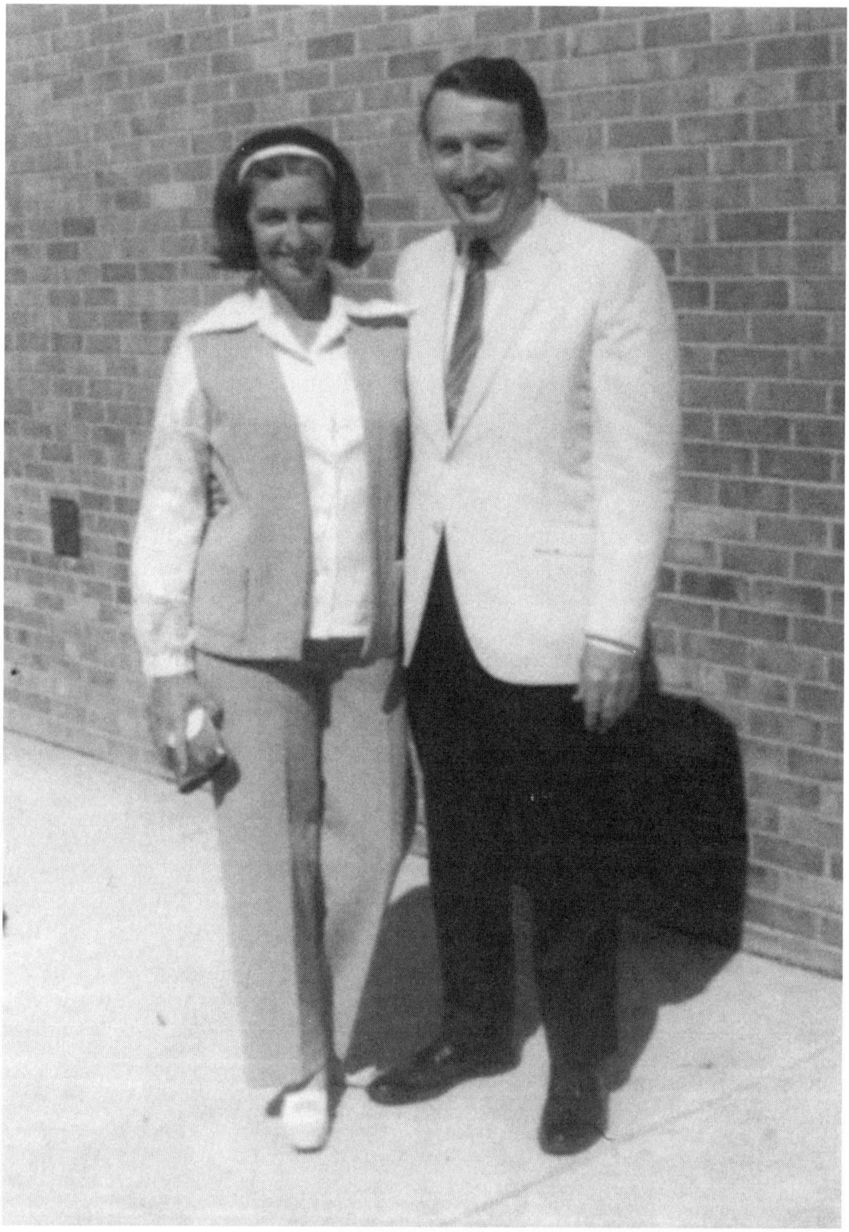

1950: Dale and Betty Bumpers, young married couple, Chicago

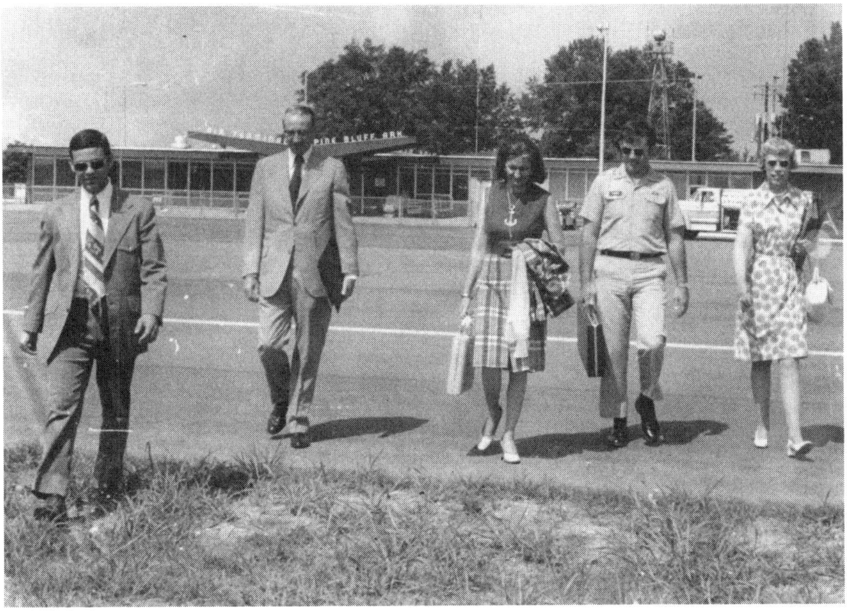

Immunization Planning Team: Every Child in 1973 with John Bailey, security, AR State Police; Dr. Runyon Deere, USDA; Betty Bumpers, First Lady of Arkansas; Bill Lawson, AR National Guard; and Mary Lou Butler, Public Health, Department of Nursing

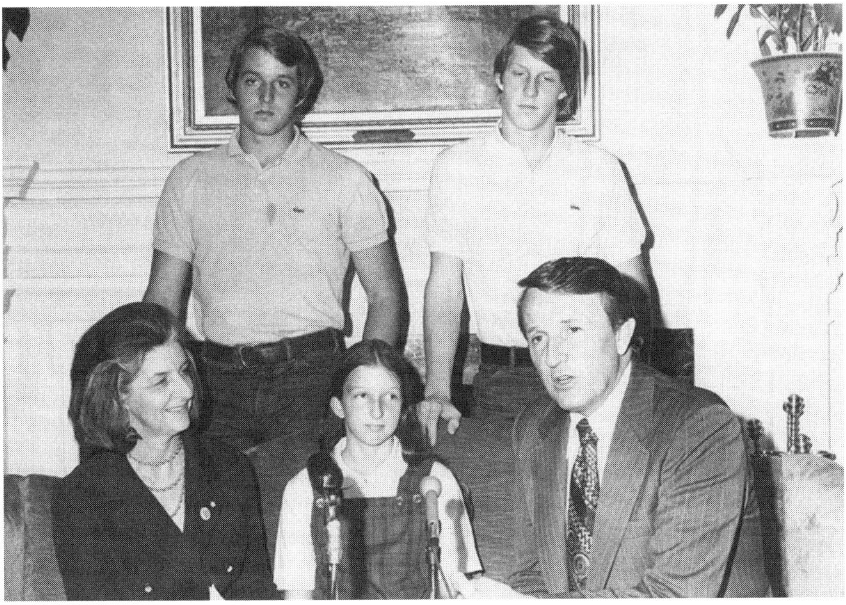

Immunization Press Conference: Bumpers family (*Courtesy of the UALR Center for Arkansas History and Culture*)

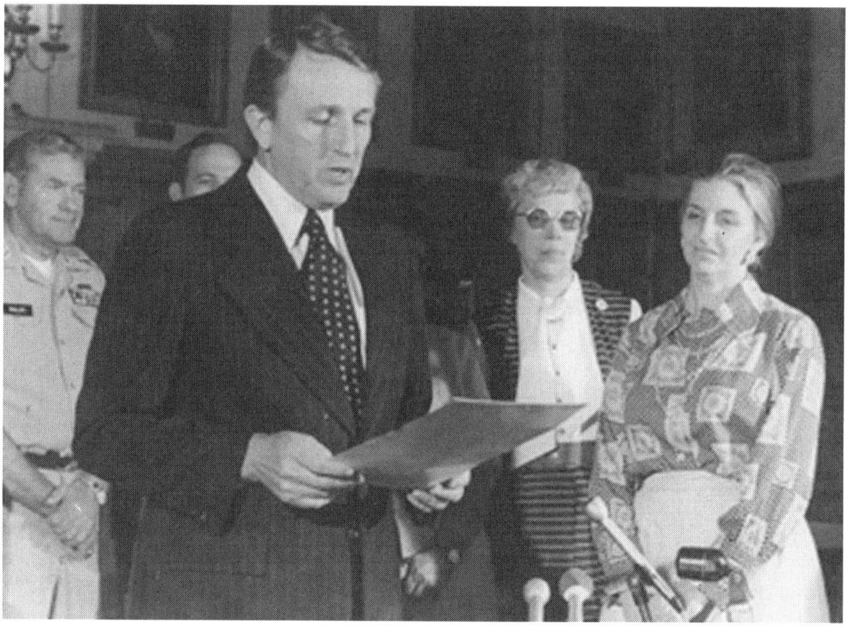

Immunization Proclamation: Dale Bumpers and Betty Bumpers (*Courtesy of the UALR Center for Arkansas History and Culture*)

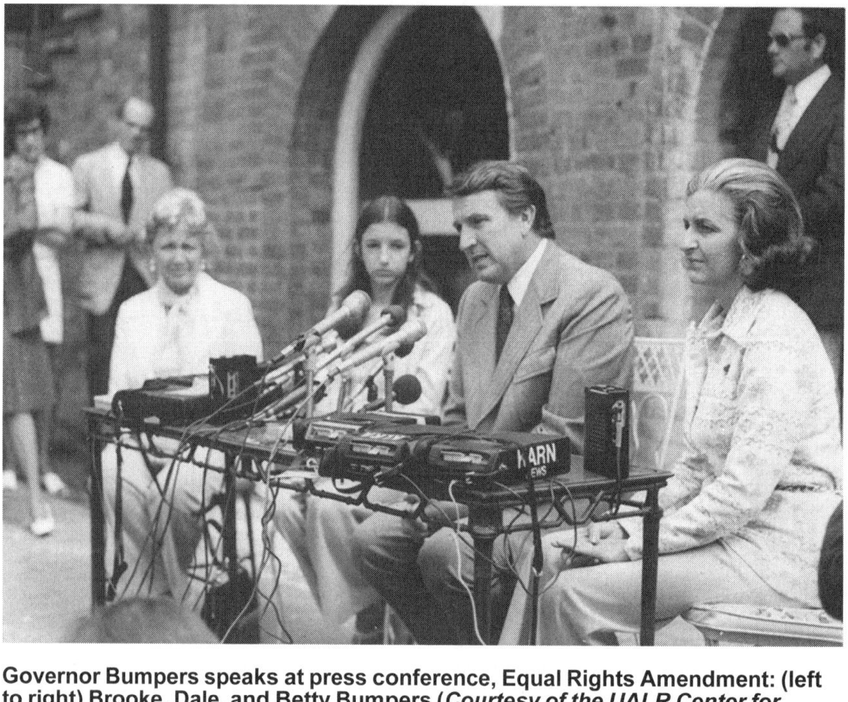

Governor Bumpers speaks at press conference, Equal Rights Amendment: (left to right) Brooke, Dale, and Betty Bumpers (*Courtesy of the UALR Center for Arkansas History and Culture*)

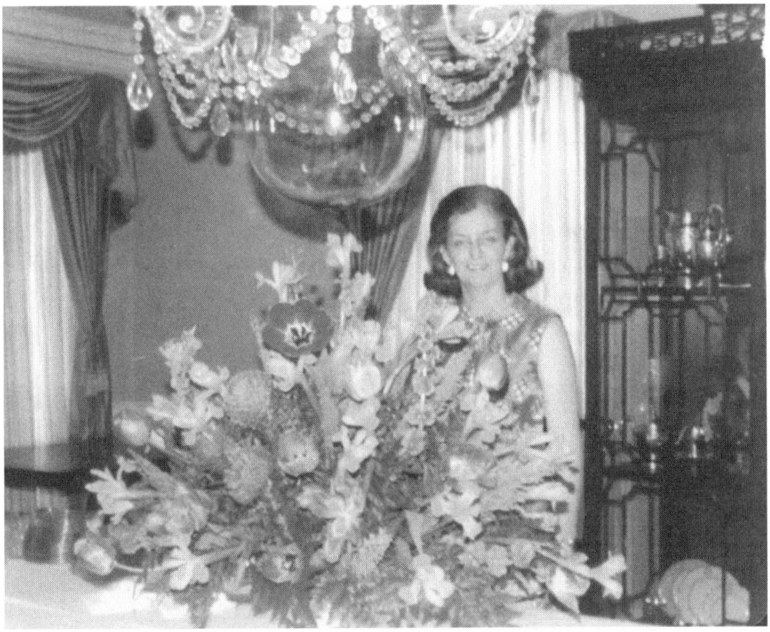

Betty Bumpers, governor's mansion, 1973

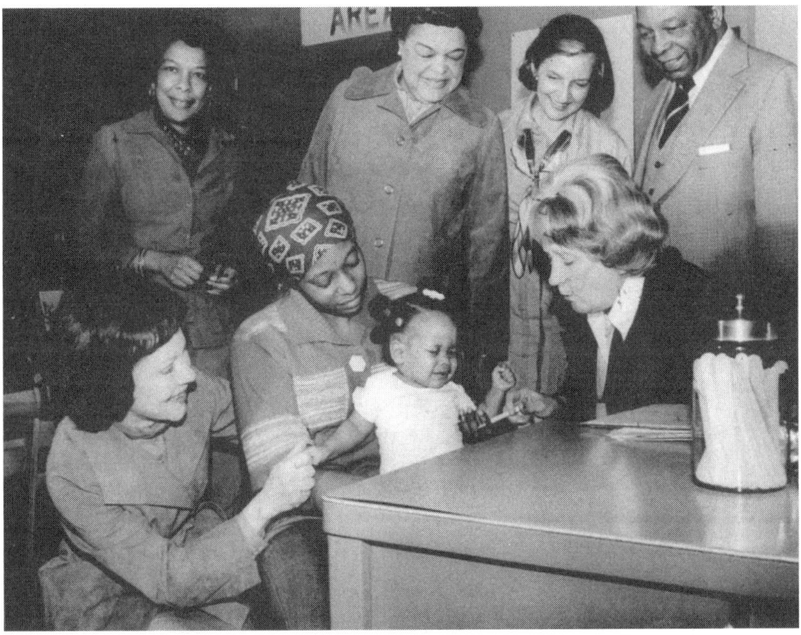

"World Health Day, 1975," national "kick off" of combined vaccines. Back row: Dr. Roz Epps, D.C. Dept. of Health; Bettena Washington; Betty Bumpers; Walter Washington, mayor of D.C. Front row: First Lady Rosalynn Carter; a parent; child; and Public Health nurse

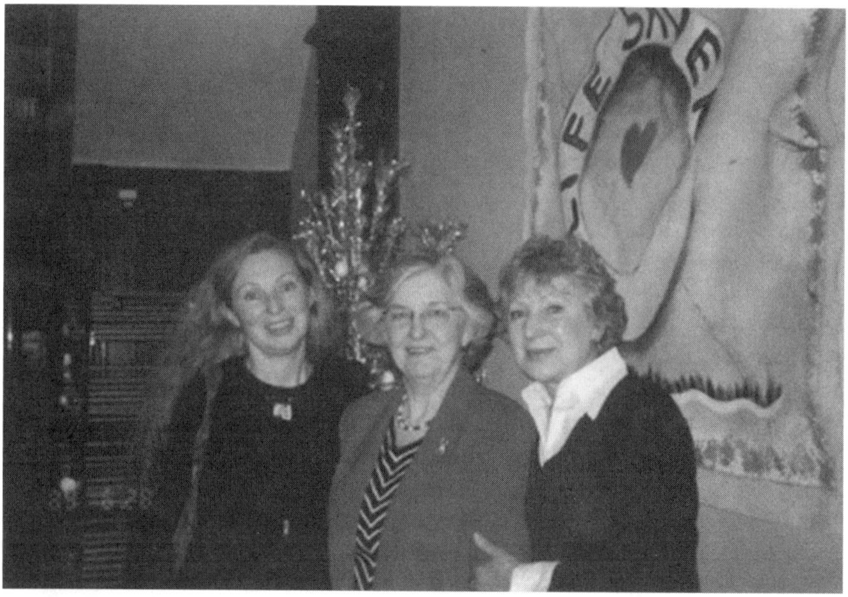

Larissa, Betty, and Lala Cornelius (Larissa's daughter) (*Courtesty of Larissa Skuratovskaya*)

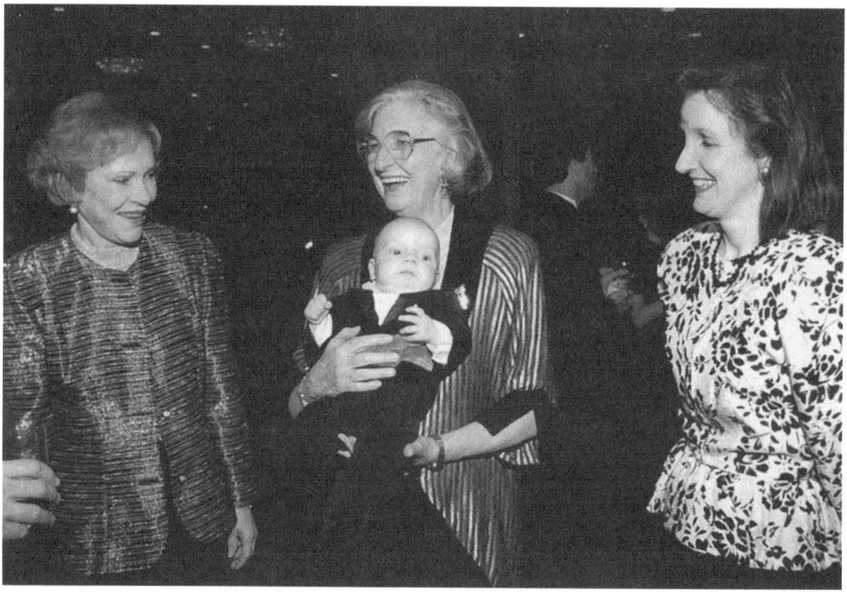

Peace Links Gala: First Lady Rosalynn Carter, Betty Bumpers with grandson Callan Low, and daughter Brooke Bumpers Low

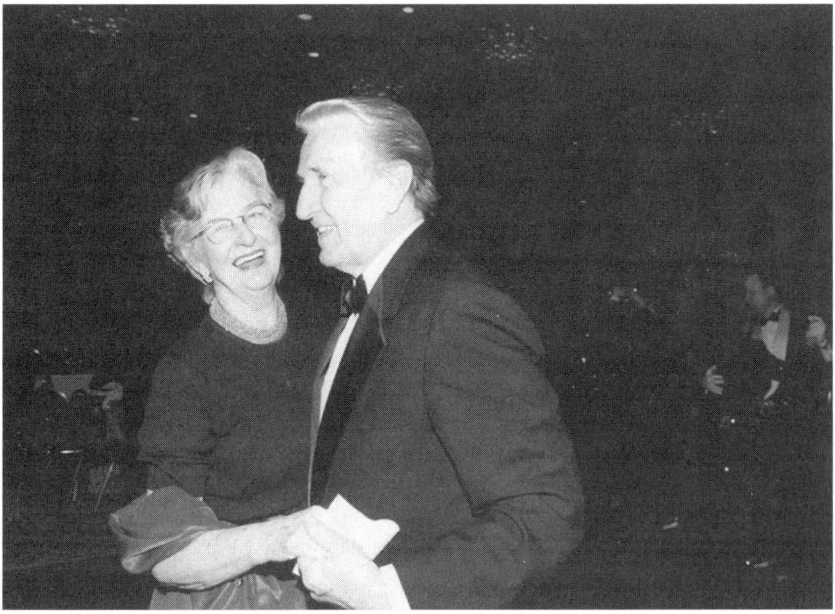

Peace Links Gala: Dancing with Dale and Betty Bumpers

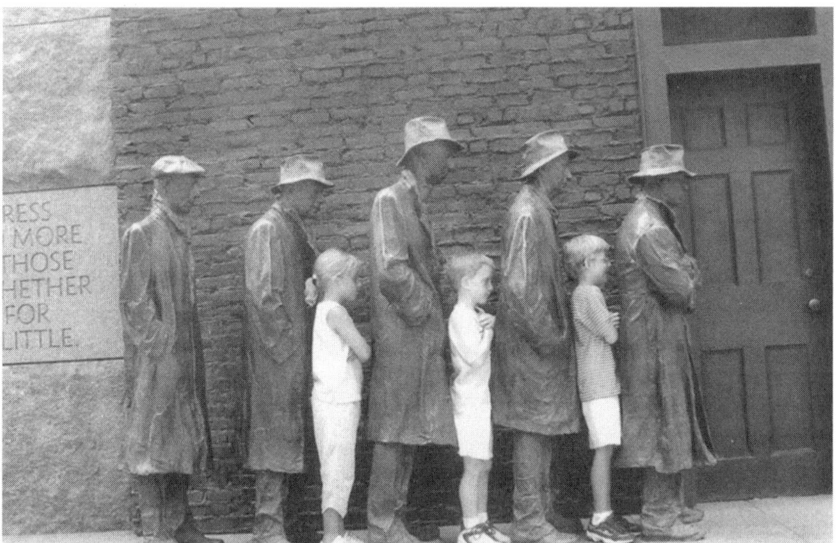

Grandchildren at FDR Memorial: Meg Bumpers, Callan Low, and Alex Bumpers

SIX

Marrying, Creating a Family, and Volunteering

> I tell my kids never to shrink from any experiences because somewhere down the road in your life, you will use the experience. It may be fifty years from the time you learned it, but it will be information that you use.

CONVERSATIONS WITH BETTY

Dale and I had been courting for about nine years, and we had become engaged. We had made a commitment to marry, though we hadn't set a date. Dale had started at Northwestern University Law School in September, and in March, during his second semester, his parents were killed in a car wreck. Dale left school and came back to Charleston to settle his parents' estate. He stayed home while his brother, Carroll, went back to a yearlong program he was in at Harvard. His sister, Margaret, went back to her vending business in Ohio. I went ahead and finished out the year at University of Arkansas.

After he lost his parents, Dale and I decided we would get married late that summer of 1949, and we had our wedding in September. Then we moved to Chicago, and Dale went back to law school. I went back to The Fair Store and got a part-time job. Dale had the GI Bill, of course, but we needed the money I made. Dale wanted to go home to Charleston practically every weekend because his dad had left several different businesses, and Dale needed to see to them.

We enjoyed spending holidays in Charleston because Ruth and Maggie and their husbands lived there; it was home to us. Bequita was still single, but she was nearby, working in Fort Smith. Bernice was in Missouri, and we would stop on the way pretty often to see her and her husband. Because of our traveling, I had several different jobs at The Fair Store that fall. But I was so bored, I was about to go out of my mind. Selling curtains was my first job. Then I started selling hats because of contacts I'd made when I was at the school of design.

I liked part-time work because it let us spend vacations with my mother and dad—we would drive there and just move in during our breaks. We were somehow more tied to my parents because Dale had lost his. It was like an umbilical cord—we'd come home for vacations, and I would just quit my job. Or I would say, "I'm going home, I've got to go home. I'm going to be gone for two weeks," and I would just leave. Then, one time, The Fair Store wouldn't let me off, so I had to quit. When I went back after Christmas, I got another job through an employment agency.

That job was with Reliance Manufacturing, and I worked with two designers on dresses and other clothes. I would draft and cut the patterns for them, then cut out and make the sample dresses. I was excited about the work because one of the designers did dresses for Nelly Dawn. I remember that my mother had one or two Nelly Dawn dresses; they were not really cheap but nice, kind of middle-line expensive.

Another designer did dresses for J. C. Penney; I think the line was called the Happy Home. J. C. Penney bought a lot of dresses and demanded more quality, so we had to add things because of the volume of orders they bought. I would add a quarter of an inch to the seam allowances, and they didn't want little cheap plastic belts. Instead, we made self-belts out of the dress fabric; they were long and tied in a bow or a knot. The sweep of the skirt had to be wider, so I would add eight inches to the samples that we showed and sold to J. C. Penney. That was a fun, exciting job. I kept it a good while, and Dale and I would still come home to Charleston every vacation time.

Because Reliance Manufacturing let me off, I kept working for them for about a year and a half and held three different jobs. I kept working while Dale went to school in the summer. Even though they were lenient about letting me off for breaks, I felt bad about leaving so much. Also, it was hard to get there on the subway, and I had to ride it home all alone.

Then I heard about a job at Passavant Hospital, near where Dale was in school. Northwestern's law, business, and medical schools are on the downtown campus, not out in Evanston. This hospital was right next to the downtown campus, and I applied to be a librarian. This was a great job because Passavant was *the* hospital in Chicago. It was prestigious, and all the wealthy people went there. It was considered a privilege to die there.

The hospital had a beautiful little library, mainly for the staff and the doctors but also for patients. The library got fabulous collections from people because Mrs. Armor and Mrs. Swift, of the meatpacking businesses, were both on the hospital's auxiliary board. They also were the ones who did the debutante ball in Chicago. In fact, as board members, they both, along with Mrs. Davis, [former First Lady] Nancy Reagan's mother, interviewed me for the job and hired me to operate that library. The chief of staff at the hospital was Dr. Loyal Davis, Nancy Reagan's stepfather.

The hospital had a French chef, and we could eat at a great discount. So when Dale finished for the day, he would come over and we would have dinner. Then he would go next door and study at the law library. That's when I started my life of volunteerism; I started working with brain surgery patients. Loyal Davis was a neurosurgeon, and he was doing early brain surgery. These patients had to relearn things because the surgery traumatized their brains. So that's how I started; I volunteered to teach the patients basic reading skills and help them to recover.

All day, I took a cart with books, candy, and so on around to the patients' rooms. Sometimes Mrs. Armor, Mrs. Swift, and Mrs. Davis also volunteered. They would get big donations of books, a whole collection from some prestigious library or from someone who had died. Then, after Dale and I ate dinner, I would continue working at the library, cataloging books. Mrs. Davis, especially, would come in and help me because her husband was there operating, putting in long, long hours. She'd stay and hang out, reading or cataloging, and we became great friends. She also worked in the coffee shop, a real Miss Volunteer, a Miss Candy Striper.

When Dale finished studying for the night, he'd come over and get me, and we'd drive home. We lived out toward Evanston, and our apartment was right across the street from the elevated-train track. The back of the apartment was on the alley. It was cheap, but the location was great. The first time my sister Maggie and brother-in-law stayed with us, this really fast train came through in the middle of the night. We had been talking and talking, and she hadn't paid much attention to the noise, except for two or three times. They had just gone to bed when this train came through. She jumped out of bed and came running in and said, "Jesus God, what was that?"

But we got used to it. We didn't sleep in the bedroom, where we'd put them. We slept on a Murphy bed that dropped down from the wall in the living room, where we didn't hear the train as much. We fought a lot at that time; we needed time to adjust. Both of us were working, and it was hard with his studying and all. We used to get into the screams on the way home, and if I hadn't been so far from Charleston, with so much time to kill, I probably would've gone back there. But that was a great job; the hospital graciously let me off at spring break to come home, and Dale and I would drive that thousand miles from Chicago to Charleston, sometimes nonstop. So we made it through. I worked at the library until Dale graduated, and then we moved back to Charleston.

Dale's brother Carroll had married, and his wife wanted to go to California. She didn't want to live in Arkansas because, in the hot summertime, she was one of those women who flushed red. She hated the hot weather, so they took off after Carroll graduated from Harvard. Dale and Carroll graduated at the same time. They both had been in the service, and though Carroll was a year ahead of Dale, he had dropped out because he had to take rabies shots and then developed complications. During those years—that was the early 1950s—lawyers were having a tough time. They couldn't find jobs. Carroll and his wife ended up in Redwood City, California, where he worked for Standard Oil in San Francisco.

In the meantime, Dale was looking for a job; we just didn't know what to do. Dale decided to buy back his father's hardware and furniture store, which had been sold while settling the estate. His dad had owned a frozen-food locker plant that they developed right after World War II, and he had a hardware and furniture store where he had worked during the Depression. It sold machinery—all kinds of farm equipment, nails, wire, and barbed wire—as well as appliances.

Dale's father had first worked at the store, and then he bought into it. He owned it along with a partner, a younger person who was a really good mechanic and had started as a bicycle repairman. The partner was a genius with all kinds of small machinery, and Dale's father took care of the books. Though he knew that the partner didn't have a strong business sense, he had never said that to Dale, so Dale didn't know. Dale's dad was one of those very strict people who never said anything bad about anybody. Consequently, his children knew nothing about the realities of a lot of people. Of course, Dale has always been the boy who has to learn the hard way.

Dale's father had left instructions that if anything happened to him, they should just get rid of the hardware business. But the partner asked Dale to buy the store. Dale knew I wanted to stay in Charleston because all of my family—and a lot of his, too—were there. Back then, young lawyers who set up practice on their own were not paid well. So Dale did buy the store. He was always so bullheaded, you couldn't tell him anything, but that's what made him a successful lawyer and a good governor and senator, I guess.

It ended up that Dale and I spent fifteen years practically as paupers because of that decision. I had to teach school, and, as Dale would say, nobody but my family knew how poor we were, except him and the banker. Dale always thought he was smart, but he didn't know some things about people. When he was young, his family talked poor. Dale's mother thought they were going to perish the next day, starve to death. So he had grown up with more insecurity about things like this than I did because I never knew I was poor when we were growing up.

Dale's parents would never say anything bad about anybody, partly because they were sanctimonious. That was good because Dale was raised with everything black and white. I was raised that way too, to some degree, but there was a little more gray area in our family, like cussing and other things. Dale's dad had never let him work in the store because he wanted him to be educated, to be a lawyer, a politician. Dale's dad had been a state legislator for two terms and thought that being a politician was a great calling, a noble profession, and he wanted Dale to serve that way. Dale would go to the courthouse steps to be there when his dad introduced all these different politicians. As a boy, Dale had delivered the newspaper, and he would have long conversations with several politicians and other people who were really interested in the news. So he was connected to the world of politics early on.

I taught elementary school for a total of five years in Charleston. I had as many as fifty-three kids in a class. The average class size was about forty, and it was so exhausting when I had so many more. I'd never sit down from the time I walked into the classroom till the time I went home at four o'clock. But thank God, we had this good principal who would help me.

When I taught art, it was considered a free period. It was noisy, and it was free, but I got reprimanded several times by different superintendents. They'd come by, hear my classroom, come in, and see these kids working under the table or up on top of the table or out under a shade tree. The superintendent would ask about it, and I would say I had sent the kids out there because it was so warm inside. In reading classes, I would divide the class up into seven or eight tables, depending on their reading level. I'd test them and then seat them. I put kids at the tables who could teach reading or spelling to the others. I'd send one of these smart kids out under the shade tree with those who couldn't read. The good readers would read stories, and the kids who couldn't would act out the stories. Then they'd come back to the classroom and put on a play. Boy, they thought they were hot spit. So teaching meant trying to do the very best with whatever I had in hand.

I was teaching school that first year back in Charleston when I got pregnant with Brent. But in those days, they wouldn't let teachers be pregnant—I couldn't show. Thank goodness the style was for little dresses with peplums. My mother helped me make a couple with peplums, which covered up the fact until I got through the school year.

I taught again the next year, thanks to Huhu. I was so fortunate that Hennie, or Huhu, as we called her, came along when Brent was born. She was a widow without children of her own, and she had been a babysitter for a friend of mine while the friend was in college. Huhu came to stay with me for a week to help with the baby, and that started the relationship with her. You had to get somebody in because you lay in bed for twelve days after the birth, and then you were so weak, you couldn't take care of the baby for a week afterwards. I was able to do some of it, though, because I wouldn't stay in the bed all those twelve days. We started using Huhu to help me out and to babysit because Dale and I tried to go out to dinner one night a week.

Bequita had married, and we would meet her and her husband, Miller, one or two nights a month. He had a hardware store in Vian, Oklahoma. We would meet in Fort Smith, which was about the same distance from Vian as from Charleston. We'd go to some inexpensive café, have dinner, and maybe see a movie. Hennie would come and babysit, then, after I had my second baby, she came more often. It was hard to scrape together enough money to pay her, but we didn't have to pay a lot. She also worked as a telephone switchboard operator.

As Hennie didn't have any family nearby, it was kind of a mutual thing when she came to us. She adopted us as her family, and we adopted her as ours, so it was ideal. It was a lifelong commitment, just as though we truly had adopted each other. She helped me raise my kids, and I took care of her longer than she took care of me. Hennie was very gregarious and sweet, and she had been lonely. She loved us, and when she got to where she said, "I don't care if you pay me or not," Dale immediately started making Social Security payments on her wages because he knew it would give her a good retirement; we just paid her a token amount a lot of times.

Hennie took up living with us and went on every vacation with us. She was like my mother, except my mother was too busy helping Maggie with her four kids. My mother was also running her own household and taking care of my dad, and, at her age, she didn't particularly want to babysit. I understood that, and I didn't want to impose on her.

Huhu was the only babysitter my kids ever knew. She took care of Brent while I taught, both the first year after he was born and again the next year. At the end of the second year, when he was eighteen or nineteen months old, I came home from school one day and said, "Well, honey what have you and Huhu done all day?"

He said, "Well, we warrrshed and we arrrrned. I hepped [helped]."

Here he was, speaking like his babysitter, copying even bad grammar and things like that. I thought, "What am I doing teaching school, teaching other children and not raising my own?" At that time I was pregnant with Bill, and I was going through the same thing to disguise the fact. I got by with it for both of them because Bill was an August baby, and Brent was born in October. The school had the pregnancy policy so the kids wouldn't know that a teacher "did that." Like the kids could even relate to it! But that's typical school board stuff; think how far we have progressed.

I quit teaching school the year Bill was born. I made that commitment to stay home and raise my children, and it was the hardest thing I ever did. It was hard because there are lots of boring hours in rearing children, and you have to make a real commitment because it's tough work. As my kids came along, I took them places, made time for them, and disciplined myself to stay home. A lot of child rearing is especially boring if you have had an exciting job. I loved teaching, and I loved the work world; it's easier than staying at home. Most people think stay-at-home mothers have the easiest job in the world, but they don't. It's like anything else; to get anything to pay off, you have to work hard, and then success comes. I loved rearing my family. I loved raising my kids and watching them learn.

We spent eighteen years in Charleston after we married. I had grown up thinking I had to put three meals a day on the table, and my husband was home for lunch every day for those eighteen years. We lived within three blocks of Dale's hardware store and the law office, my mother lived close by, and so did my sister Maggie. Later, Maggie and I built new houses and lived right next door to each other.

Dale and the fellows would get up early for work and have breakfast in town with friends, or Dale would go there and read the newspaper while he ate. My mother used to think it was terrible that I didn't get up and fix his breakfast or that he didn't stay home for it. I said, "I don't blame him. I wish I could go to town and have breakfast and read the paper." He did that maybe two or three days a week, but I always made lunch and cooked dinner at night. We were working our tushes off. I had a garden and did canning, and I was helping my mother with her great big old garden because mine wasn't that big. I also mowed my own yard. I did a little bit of everything and volunteered for things; I was PTA health officer for fifteen years.

But mostly, I was a stay-at-home mother. We were busy with Maggie's family; she'd had three boys in less than three years—bing, bing, bing—and another later. We did a lot of stuff together. We belonged to a square dance club and did some dancing. In Charleston we also had a little country club with a public golf course where I used to play before Brooke was born. I don't remember who furnished the money for it, but there was some sort of grant to establish golf courses for small towns. Each course would serve maybe five communities; ours was called the County Line Country Club.

We started getting too busy. Along with teaching, the kids, and volunteering, I was in a garden club and did the flowers for the church every Sunday. I grew a lot in my yard, and I had cadres of women who would call when they had some pretty flowers in their gardens. So my weekends were full, and in our spare time, we did things with the garden club to beautify the city. We planned and planted; the magnolia trees and some of our other plantings are still there.

Dale was working hard trying to pull that hardware business up, and we still weren't so well off financially. We were just part of the working class. Except when Dale was occupied with choir practice on Wednesday nights, he worked. The store was open on Saturday nights until eight or nine o'clock, depending on how much business they were doing, and then sometimes he opened early on Sunday morning. Dale has never been a big socializer—because he worked too hard.

The store sold television sets, and that meant he had to install them. A lot of people are too young to remember, but every house with a television set had to have an antenna. He put up practically all of the TV antennas in Charleston; he'd climb up ladders onto the roofs of houses all over town and install those antennas and the guide wires that held them. Those TVs and that hardware store were our life's bread and butter.

Sometimes he would have to drive to Fort Smith later in the day if he had a hearing for a lawsuit he was handling. Two or three times in the wintertime he rushed home and didn't even bathe. If he had time, he would put on a suit and tie, and I would drive him to Fort Smith while he worked on his brief. A time or two he forgot to change his shoes—he was all dressed up in a suit and still had on the tennis shoes he wore to climb up on roofs. We had to turn around and go back for his dress shoes.

We stayed connected to politics. We always voted, like my dad always voted, as a yellow dog Democrat. I knew Dale had been introduced early to politics by his father, but I didn't know that Dale was going to be a politician, even after we married and moved back to Charleston. I knew it by the time he ran for the Arkansas House, but he lost that one.

After I had Brooke, I zeroed in on my family. We had lost my brother young. He had been a heavy smoker, and he had a heart attack and died at age forty-two. He left six children for my mom and dad to help raise and educate. We were all working hard because times were tough, and then Brooke got sick.

Brooke and I are very close, and if you knew her medical history, you would know why. She developed a spinal tumor when she was eighteen months old. She had to have surgery, and she spent some birthdays in the hospital. The first surgery in the hospital at Fort Smith left her victimized by the medical profession. I'm grateful for the smart pediatrician who guided us on to Children's Hospital Boston instead of treating her with radiation, which could have paralyzed her.

I think she was about nine months old when she manifested the first symptoms, although we didn't recognize them. She was just not a well child. She was irritable, and she wouldn't sit up straight in her high chair. So I fed her until she was practically two because she didn't like the mess from the food coming down her arm or onto her dress.

I started noticing that she staggered sometimes when she walked, and she would fall down more often than she had when she first started walking. When we got her into the doctor, he did the pediatrician's thing of running the end of the little hammer they use to test reflexes up the bottoms of her feet. One foot reacted differently from the other, so he knew there was a problem; the X-ray showed that her spine was blocked. This was when she was almost two years old, and they decided to operate. Her surgeon was just a regular adult neurosurgeon, not used to treating children. In the operation, he left the dura [outer covering of the spinal cord] where the tumor bulged out, which was wise, but he should have left it wider open.

After the surgery, the surgeon didn't seem to have any recourse other than to use radiation. He had gathered information, and his decision was to radiate the tumor. So the surgeon talked to me a little bit about how, if she were older and had been walking, they might consider something else. I didn't understand what he was saying, that we might consider some other recourse. It might be more traumatic, he said, but as young as she was, she wouldn't even remember having walked. She had just had her birthday in the hospital, her second birthday.

Our pediatrician had been at Duke and was very skilled. He had come back to his hometown to set up his pediatric practice, and he monitored the situation and watched over Brooke. I realized it was something grave that the radiation would do, so I told the pediatrician that he would have to make the decision, that we just couldn't make that kind of decision ourselves. He took the next step and got the surgeon's report and the pathology report. Then he called Children's Hospital Boston and talked to them about it, and they told him that radiation would not kill the tumor. It was a low-grade tumor, which means it didn't have much vascular system. The radiation would do nothing but destroy the spinal cord, and she would be left a paraplegic.

Our pediatrician arranged for us to go to Children's Hospital Boston and see Dr. Maxton, who worked with brain tumors. He was a pediatric neurosurgeon, which was a new specialty. Dr. Maxton was bringing in neurosurgeons from all over the world to train them. So we took her to Boston, and he did an evaluation of her and told us to take her home and watch her carefully. He stayed in touch with our pediatrician and our local family doctor.

So anytime something unusual happened with her, we would worry. I didn't know at the time that they were worried about problems that would affect her renal system, but still she recovered. Then she developed a nerve twitch in her side that was like neuralgia. She would be running and playing, and all of a sudden, she would act like something was paining her. Finally, when she got to the point that she couldn't sleep well, they had to do something. I sat up many, many nights in front of the fireplace with her stretched across a big pillow on my lap, with her head kind of hanging off one side of the chair and her feet off the other. She also could sleep if she was stretched out, and I just walked the floor with her head on my shoulder and her back stretched down, which added space in her spinal cord.

Finally, just before she was four, all of the doctors, including the local doctor and the pediatrician, told us to take her to Boston for surgery. So we did, and they did nine laminectomies, procedures on the support bones of the back. They removed nine of those bones—that knob that sticks out on your back. They clipped those nine bones and threw them away. [Lamina may be removed to allow access to the spinal canal.][1] They also did a stripping operation of the tumor, and fortunately it worked. They got lucky. They got 90 percent of the tumor, and they believed if they could get the eye of a tumor like that, it would die. We didn't know for two years whether they had got it, but it became clear that they had.

She was doing wonderfully; she was in physical therapy and doing well. Then, suddenly, she got a very high fever, and it turned out she had meningitis associated with debris from the surgery. Thank goodness they did spinal taps to make sure it wasn't viral meningitis, which it wasn't. She couldn't walk for a while, and the physical therapy stopped, too. It was a dreadful time. We don't know how much damage was done by the surgery, by the meningitis, or by the lack of early physical therapy.

Brooke took up much of my time after that surgery. She wore a leather and steel body brace that kept her growing straight. She had to relearn how to walk, which took a long time, and I had to do physical therapy with her four times a day to keep the muscles working. Once you let muscle atrophy, it can never be brought back. It takes a long time to learn physical therapy, and I had to do it right to keep all of the muscles alive, especially in her right leg. We took her back to Boston every six months to make sure that I was exercising all the muscles so they would stay viable. Those were trying years. Because nerves are the slowest-growing tissue in the body, the doctors told me recovery would take up to two years.

And I remember the day when she said she was better. I would do these exercises with her toes, to turn them under, and she would work on pushing them for a long time, forcing them down, until she finally knew how to do it. I would say, "Turn your toes under. Up, down, up, down; ten times." And then, "Turn your foot this way." I had to get her to exercise every muscle. One day almost two years later, she turned her toes in and said, "Mommy, I can feel my toes."

Still, we had to do physical therapy at least once a day, to keep stretching, until she reached her maximum growth at about sixteen. One of Brooke's legs is highly sensitive and weak, and the other one is sort of numb but muscular and helps her walk. So physical therapy is important; it keeps that weak leg stretched out so that it doesn't pull up tight and cause her to limp badly. She has let it go for a while, but she gets back into therapy and keeps it minimized.

So Brooke and I have had a very—I don't know what you'd call it—symbiotic relationship. If I ever did anything successful in my life, it was raising a handicapped daughter who didn't know she was handicapped. She's all right, and she hasn't paid that much attention to it, she has been so busy with her life.

Of course, in her childhood, everyone was very attentive to Brooke because she was fragile, she was in a brace, and for two or three years we had thought we were going to lose her. She was the only girl in the family aside from my sister Ruth's daughter, and they lived in Fort Smith. Brooke was the only girl in the neighborhood, and she grew up with about nine boys who all took care of her. She would get out and play football with them, but they knew to watch her and be careful. They all kind of pampered and petted her. The kids had this very creative first cousin who was close by, one of my sister's boys. He was just a little older than my oldest child, and he loved Brooke. He spent a lot of time with me because his father was sort of verbally rough on him. The boy was one of those worriers who would wring his hands. He was artistic, and I encouraged that.

Because my daughter couldn't get away from home easily, I had friends in to play with her. By listening to their play, I picked up on the fact that she was becoming a bully. It was her territory, so when they played doctor, she was always the doctor; she would call the parameters. So I really went to work on how that's not the way to do things. I told her that it is not right for you to play that way just because the other kids are in your house. I listened a lot while my kids played. When the boys were back in their room, I would be in the bathroom right next to it, listening. You pick up on whether they're playing fair, whether they're bullying, and whether they're into something they shouldn't be into.

Holidays were not as big a deal in those days. We had great birthday parties for all of our kids until they were twelve, and then I said, "No more birthday parties; you are on your own." We still don't do anything except call and wish each other a happy birthday. Our holiday activities centered on the community because I was involved in so many things. We always had a Christmas parade, and I would help at school. We would do a float with my class during the time I was teaching.

On Christmas we always went to my mother and dad's house. My grandmother had died while I was in college, so we didn't go to her house like we did when I was a young child. We had gone there for Christmas and Easter or to my grandparents' in Branch, but they had died as well. At Easter, while my kids were young, we were busy in the church. The choir always did an Easter cantata, and I entertained them with a dinner party after the special performances.

The church was just part of the community and part of our social life when we were young. After we married and moved back, the church was still our social life. Dale's father had taught a Sunday school class called the Bumpers's Class for Young Married Couples, though it included older people. There was also a Sunday school class for older men and another for ladies. Dale took over his dad's class after we came back from Chicago and he had graduated and married. He taught the class for eighteen years. He had to study every Saturday night or during the week after work or get up early Sunday morning to prepare.

Dale talked about our Methodist church in his book. He referred to me a time or two as just a "Sunday school girl who met the Sunday school boy," and that kind of stuck with us. When asked, "Where do you get your guiding principles?" he would say, "I met this Sunday school girl." We were taught church literature and given guidelines, and we had some wonderful ministers in Charleston. It has always been a progressive town with a very active Methodist church.

The Methodist church tends to change ministers quite often, and Charleston would get either young ministers who were on their way up or older ministers who had been district superintendents. We were fortunate; we got a lot of very intelligent, good men. I remember one minister who came there after Dale and I were married but before I was pregnant with Brent. The minister said, "You know, this is the first church I have ever served that does not have a nursery. You know and I know that several young couples here need to get on with the business of starting their families." The next year, he christened eight babies.

A couple of years later, one of those families lost a baby. The minister had been moved to another church not very far from us. He was a wise old man and sweet, but he was fragile and frequently sick and needed a less active church. The mother asked our old minister if he would come back and preach at her baby's funeral. She was a friend of mine, and I had gone along with her. He said, "You know, one of the things that has held me in good stead all my life is that I have always tried to practice good manners. In the Methodist church, the minister is not your church. So it would just be good manners for you to let your preacher preach that funeral." Wasn't that a wonderful lesson? My friend understood it, and our new preacher did the sermon.

We became close to our ministers because we were so active in the church. Teaching Sunday school and directing the choir really fit Dale. When I fixed flower arrangements for the church, I would do two or three, depending on how available flowers were. One would be at the front and one at the entrance and maybe another on a side. I got really good at drying flowers and using them in fall arrangements. Sometimes I would mix artificial flowers in with fresh greenery and flowers. I had a collection of artificial flowers that no one ever knew were artificial. I'd use peacock feathers, too, that I got from a relative who had peacocks on his farm. Sometimes they drop beautiful feathers, and I'd use these for height in the bouquets.

One time a wonderful old man in the church came over and said, "Betty, those are the most beautifulest flowers I have ever seen in my life. What in the world kind of flowers are they?" Of course, he didn't have good eyesight, and I said, "Charlie, they are peacock feathers."

And then, later on when I'd use them, he'd say, "Betty, you got those beautiful peacock flowers again. They are just the most beautifulest things I have ever seen." I never told him again that they were just feathers.

I'd go out to the prairie for other flowers. My dad had 360 acres of virgin prairie, and he left it to me when he died. I had wanted him to give it to The Nature Conservancy, but he left that for me to take care of. We sold it to The Nature Conservancy, which may sell it to the state of Arkansas. We gave the farm to the Farmland Trust, hoping they could save the property.

Out there on the prairie, I would get liatris—it's that tall, skinny purple-top that now is sold in flower shops. The long purple, fuzzy-looking poker was wonderful for the height in a flower arrangement. The liatris would bloom about the same time that hydrangeas do, so I'd have the purple-blue or pink hydrangea with that purple-top.

One Sunday, I had those in an arrangement, and the same old man recognized me and said, "Betty, I'll tell you, you're just such a marvel. I never knew those old purple-tops were good for anything except gettin' up the legs in your overalls when you're stompin' the hay in the hay baler."

I had wonderful experiences with that task for the church, and I took some flower-arranging courses and joined a garden club. I also taught vacation Bible school for two weeks every summer, and I did the reading program at the library on weekends. I would take my children along to the library, and I would have all of the children put together flannel graphs. This was an activity I had used when I was teaching. I gave each child some flannel to draw and cut out a certain character from the story. When I read their character's part of the story, they would come up front and pin their character onto a flannel background board.

I also volunteered in health work. In the 1950s and 1960s, I assisted in school clinics as a PTA health officer. A public health nurse came to the elementary schools to do student screenings, and in the middle school, we caught a lot of scoliosis in girls. Nurses also did eye exams, and we found kids who were failing in school because they couldn't see well.

I took the chairmanship of every drive, from cancer to TB to typhoid to anything people wanted to raise money for. I always took the chairman jobs—I was chairman of drives to get to know the people out in the communities, out in the rural areas, or on the edges of towns. I knew who the "hosses" were, the women who were dependable, and I would divide up the towns with the volunteers in mind. It's how I learned to organize, I guess. You see how things get done, how to get things accomplished. You learn this if you live in a small town or community and if you pay attention. The same thing can happen in a bigger community, in cities. I think learning that has been invaluable to me for doing grassroots organizing.

Actually, grassroots work is all organizing, and those are skills that nearly anybody can learn. Lots of people learn them, and that's why I say most of our real leadership comes out of small American towns. The nine original astronauts all came from small towns. Not only did they know how to accomplish things, but they also had good egos; they had good sense. Not everybody learns those skills; they have to have some innate ability to pay attention, be good observers, and be curious.[2]

NOTES

1. "Laminectomy," www.mayoclinic.com/health/laminectomy/MY00674 (accessed September 21, 2012).
2. Betty Bumpers interviews by Anna Eblen and Jennie Eblen, August 29–September 1, 2005; May 14, 2006; October 2–6, 2007; and February 24–26, 2009.

SEVEN

Joining Political Life as First Lady of Arkansas

> Somebody described Dale as the dog that caught the car. I was like the dog that caught the car, too, so we both were thinking, "What do I do with this?"
>
> CONVERSATIONS WITH BETTY

While we lived in Charleston, we stayed in contact with extended family, and we all were involved as Dale got into political life. When he ran in the primary election for governor in 1970, in the Democratic primary he had to knock off Orval Faubus, who was running for a seventh term. Then in the general election, Dale ran against Rockefeller, who was trying to get reelected. For us, Dale's campaign for governor started with Margaret (Dale's sister), and my sisters and me. Our cousin Bequita had lost her family—her husband and both of her children—in a house fire; it was tragic. Bequita adopted Dale's campaign, and later on, Dale got her an apartment and a job as a receptionist in his office. That campaign and the work she did for him saved her.

We began by going out as door knockers, canvasing south Arkansas. They sent us there because the campaign thought Dale couldn't win that area. We would get so tired; we'd go into a town and take separate streets. A lot of women stayed home then, and we'd get a good response by going door to door. I'd say, "I'm Mrs. Bumpers. Here's some literature about Dale Bumpers, and we'd appreciate it if you'd give him your consideration." Once we were giving out our literature to people in a grocery store, and I lost my temper after a long day of door knocking. A man at the store took the literature and just threw it in his basket, and some fell on the floor. I was so aggravated, I grabbed the basket and almost knocked him over. My family and Huhu took care of the kids, and I was never gone more than four days at a time.

During the campaign, I was on a radio show, and the announcer had implied that Dale was against guns or against hunting. I said, "That's the most scurrilous piece of crap that I've ever heard. I've cleaned quail Dale brought home from hunting hundreds of times. I hated the job, but I always did it. I can't tell you how many times I got up too early, when the word came out to the hunters that the ducks were on the ponds. Several times Dale brought home duck. I don't even like the taste of it, but I'd clean the ducks."

Afterward, I thought I had really ruined Dale's chances. That interview went all over the state, and Dale called me that night. It was before cell phones, so I don't know how he knew where I was, but he did. He said, "What the hell are you trying to do? That radio interview went everywhere. Are you trying to get me beat?"

In the long run, the interview helped him. People like it when you show some spirit. Mostly, we had a great time out door knocking. Bequita was along, and the campaign distracted her from her loss. She laughed again for the first time since her husband and children had died. We had fun, and I was probably more involved in the governor's campaign than I was in any of the other campaigns.

When Dale was inaugurated as governor, the gown I wore was my sister's dress. I'd already bought one, but we thought hers would be more appropriate. So I wore it, and that inaugural gown is in the Old State House Museum in Little Rock. The exhibit has a listening stand, and in the video, I talk about the inauguration, life as First Lady, and other work I did. The museum also has my wedding dress and our wedding pictures and more about Dale as governor.

After Dale was elected governor, here I was. It wasn't that we were hometown hillbillies or anything; we'd just been in Charleston for years and had lived a very simple life. I was not an unsophisticated person, but I was also not a well-traveled person. I had been away to college, in Chicago for one year in school and then for three years while Dale was in law school, and I had worked in jobs. But we had never done any overseas traveling, except for a trip to Acapulco that Dale won once. I was not familiar with the demands of the position because he had not been in an elective office before. And there we were, the governor and First Lady of Arkansas. Well, I was sort of thinking, "What do I do?"

No one taught you how to do it—how to be the First Lady. The cook, Liza Ashley, had been there for years, and she knew how to entertain—how to fix meals and get supplies we needed. Thank God, Liza was there. She published a book with the University of Arkansas Press: *Thirty Years at the Mansion.* She wrote about the governors she had served under, and she knew the routine of what the other First Ladies had done. She had started with the Fabuses, and she had learned a lot from the chef who came there with Governor and Mrs. Rockefeller. She had really kept up, and she was a smart woman. If it hadn't been for Liza, I don't know what I would have done; it would have been so much more difficult.

I had decided to have every state senator and representative over to dinner to get personally acquainted. Every night for a week or so, we had ten guests for dinner. Like my mother would say, it's just good manners. We entertained ten at a time until we'd had the entire Arkansas House of Representatives and Senate for dinner. Once a year, we'd entertain the state supreme court justices. We wanted to know who they were and be on good terms with them. At governors' conferences, the wives talked together about these kinds of things, but no one teaches you what to do.

Winthrop Rockefeller had been a very popular governor at first, but he was a Republican, and the state legislature was Democratic. He wasn't a very effective leader, but he did a lot of planning to modernize the state. He had think tanks, like the Brookings Institution, do studies for restructuring government agencies, but he couldn't get the plans through the legislature. Rockefeller died shortly after Dale defeated his bid for another term as governor. As governor, Dale was able to get Rockefeller's restructuring plans through because they were good ideas. I know that some political scientists cited Dale as Arkansas's best governor because of that accomplishment.

The governor's mansion site was originally the Arkansas School for the Blind, which was the only school for the blind west of the Mississippi. I think the magnolia in the yard has been there as long as the school. When we moved there, I put Brooke in school at Trinity Episcopal Church because it was so close to the mansion. Her friend lived nearby, so they could play. When we were here, the mansion had a little picket fence around it, not the security fence that is there now. Dale asked the state police who were on the grounds to wear civilian clothes instead of uniforms.

I didn't know much about decorating, and the Rockefellers had just had the mansion done, so I didn't change anything inside during the first term. I left everything Mrs. Rockefeller had remodeled the way it was because she'd brought in a New York decorator, and I couldn't see any reason to change it so soon. The mansion grounds cover seven acres, and I bought three houses close by to square off the property, just as my father taught me to square off acreage. A tornado in more recent years damaged the houses, and they have since been taken down. The tornado also blew down nine blackjack oak trees from a grove that used to be there.

When I started to furnish the mansion, I requested and received $10,000 from the legislature. I got a mahogany cabinet for the silver service that was aboard the battleship USS *Arkansas*. We commissioned the round, red carpet with a state seal for the foyer and the chandelier in the dining room. Local people did the chairs with petit point representations of the great seal and the seven different flags that have flown over Arkansas.

In the dining room, when I had a lot of guests, I'd take the table apart and use plywood extensions to make five round tables. The Louis XVI–style chandelier I bought has a big bowl underneath the crystals. One time we had a leak in the roof, and water came all the way down and dripped into that bowl. That formal dining room was for guest dinners, but we usually ate in the family dining room and kitchen on a round table with a lazy Susan. That little dining room used to have a circular staircase.

In the foyer, the rug with the Arkansas seal has recently been returned to its place after some time downstairs. Work has been done to restore the rug, which used to have a blue border, and now the state is looking for someone to make a new rug. A landing and an alcove halfway to the second floor face the entrance to the house and the foyer. It used to be curtained off, and that is where Brooke had her dollhouse. She and her friend from across the street would go up there and play. Sometimes they would sit on the stairs listening to what was going on downstairs with the grown-ups, and you could see their little feet dangling over the railing. One time Brooke threw her laundry down, and it got stuck in the foyer's chandelier.

In the parlor, we had a piano, but it wasn't a grand piano like the one there now. Bill played it, and Brooke also took piano lessons while we lived in the mansion. When the high school did *My Fair Lady*, Bill got the part of Eliza Doolittle's father, and he would play the piano and practice his singing.

In the library, a door opens into a room that used to be a guest room. There was also a guesthouse, and Eunice Shriver and Angela Lansbury stayed in the mansion's guesthouse while we were there. Holly trees used to grow outside the library window, and one of the best things I ever saw was a group of cedar waxwings there. They are pretty rare birds, and I saw them sitting in those holly bushes, eating the berries.

I tried to open the governor's mansion to the people of Arkansas. One of my secretary's tasks was to arrange tours of the mansion for schoolchildren. I had the Arkansas symphony come on the grounds, and then I'd invite the neighbors and other people from Little Rock and the area. I planted the Arkansas oaks near the gate, and I had specimen pines planted in the roundabout circle. I put in the herb garden. One of my favorite memories is looking out the bedroom window on a foggy winter night and seeing the lighted Christmas tree on top of one of the tall buildings downtown.

In Little Rock, the First Methodist Church was part of our social life, and it was one of the reasons Dale had so much support everywhere. And I mean everywhere. That was a big congregation that really supported us. It was not quite the closest church to the mansion, and during the winter we went to another one. Also, we usually came home to Charleston at least two weekends a month, so we weren't at that church in Little Rock all of the time. The church has always remained a habit—once you are in the habit of going to church every Sunday, you just go to church every Sunday. And my kids were raised in the church—they were in church every Sunday until they left home.

A lot of people in Little Rock really helped me look at the opportunities offered to me as First Lady. They helped me pick and choose and decide what to do. I wanted to be as helpful and effective as I could be, but it was difficult to sort out what would be best to do and what my real interests were.

I took up the Rockefellers' arts education ideas. Jeanette Rockefeller had come up with the concept of the Art Mobile and the idea of taking it around the state, but she hadn't put personal time into organization. The facility was ready, and I knew from living in a small town how important that service would be to people—how much children would love the arts and the plays the troupe put on.

Though the Art Mobile idea had been started, I don't remember that she did a lot with it. She was not a hands-on person, but she put money into the Arkansas Art Center and had a sophisticated level of involvement with bringing artists in. She did not go into schools like I did, as she did not have my experience of coming from a small Arkansas town and knowing the school system. She wouldn't have known how little exposure to art was offered in the schools.

The Art Mobile was languishing there at the Arkansas Art Center. So I had the idea of putting some good pieces of art in it, especially familiar pieces that we happened to have good copies of. We chose Gilbert Stuart's unfinished portrait of George Washington, which is in Boston's Museum of Fine Arts. So many duplications of the portrait were on calendars that even rural people were familiar with it, and we explained the techniques and why the portrait was unfinished. We also had Pierre-Auguste Renoir's picture of the little girl in the blue gown. We also had other art objects, and we added a recording that addressed the pictures when someone stepped in front of them.

I said, "If you educate kids or people in a community on one painting—give them some really good appreciation of one painting that they are even slightly familiar with—they suddenly become art experts, and they'll forever enjoy those pictures. They're really interested, and they will pass that word on to other people. It turns them into art lovers; it turns them into people who appreciate art. You have to educate people before they feel like they have some ownership." And people responded; they loved it. Then I got a potter who traveled with the Art Mobile and set up his wheel on the back of it. He would throw a pot and give little pieces of clay to kids just to introduce them to making pots.

The Arkansas Art Center also began other programs that Jeanette Rockefeller had set up. The children's theater put on little plays, with costumes, that were wonderfully done. A young man named Bill Bond took these plays on tour, plays like *Androcles and the Lion*, *Jack and the Beanstalk*, and many others. I talked him into doing a drama manual. I argued that all of the schools needed more information about plays, and I knew this from teaching in that little rural school and living in a small town. Theater is one thing we have in common all over the United States because every high school from a Podunk town to the most sophisticated big city has a junior-senior play. People love it, especially the students who get to participate in any part of the production, from being in the play to building the sets to doing makeup. The schools lack expertise and just draw on teachers; they call on someone and say, "You have to sponsor the play this year." Teachers typically know nothing about staging, nothing about how to put on a play. When I first had to do a pageant, I didn't know anything about stage makeup or writing down inventory or listing what you need—none of the things that go into a production.

I said, "Bill, if you would just put together layman's information about how you put on a play, it would be so helpful for the schools. It could be handed out to whichever teacher is going to sponsor that year's play. It could have simple things, like what you need to buy and how to put together a schedule for the event." So he did a workbook and illustrated it with simple hand drawings showing things like how to do staging and costuming and how to make up the eyes so they project and show to the audience. The Arkansas Art Center reproduced the manual, and it has been a wonderful aid to teachers; it is still used around the state.

My position as governor's wife gave me entrée for many of the things I did, but I also knew how to get things done: Go to the top. I started by going to superintendents of schools and selling them on the idea of bringing the Art Mobile to their schools and keeping it for three days so the public as well as the school kids could come through it. But it was a hard sell, and it was hard to get started. I had the experience of being a teacher, so I knew how to talk to them about the needs.

The Art Mobile did become successful with time, but I learned another thing by going around to the superintendents. This was right after racial integration took place, and we were trying to bring more black teachers into the schools. We had black students, but we'd torn up our educational system and turned our neighborhood schools into busing units. In a way, education was in chaos in the South. What I discovered was that lots of those superintendents ran good schools.

I suddenly realized that the reason was that they had enough sense to know that parents do not care what color a teacher is as long as their children love her and feel like they are learning. They don't care whether the teacher is purple, green, white, black, or whatever. Parents will accept those who are talented enough to be good teachers. The superintendents who knew that were the smart ones. I followed up with some of them and realized they successfully integrated their schools because they related to the parents, plus the teachers, plus the students.

I used being a governor's wife shamelessly and tried to do as much as I could. As I worked on things that little towns lacked, I was able to call on the expertise of state facilities and employees. When I started the immunization drive that later became a national model, I used the same approach and drew on local, state, and federal organizations and agencies. I used agencies like the Agricultural Extension Service because while I was growing up, I'd had experience with that and with the liberal ideas that came from Franklin Roosevelt.

Hennie [Huhu] moved into the governor's mansion with us and stayed for a year and a half. She became lonely because she didn't have much to do and was not a person who particularly enjoyed social situations. She wanted to come home to Charleston, and we were coming home practically every weekend anyway. At first, she used her parents' house, but it was out at the edge of town, so we helped her buy a nice, small house. We would do things to help her fix it up, like give her a storm window for Christmas or something like that.

Bill and Brooke were older when Hennie went back to Charleston, and Brent was away at college. Bill was with us for three of our four years in the governor's mansion and would be there with Brooke if we were gone. Linda Miesner moved in as my secretary after Hennie left. I turned over the party planning and the tours of the mansion to her. By myself, I couldn't handle all of the dinners, the parties, and the activities that I was involved in, and Linda helped. She also could babysit Brooke, and I had Liza, who cooked and helped watch Brooke later on, until Brooke was old enough not to need looking after.

I do think about how, when Brooke was sick and later when we moved to Little Rock, I kind of failed Brent, my older son. When he graduated from high school, he was just seventeen, and that was the year Dale ran for governor. Brent went off to college in the fall when he had just turned eighteen and Dale had just been elected. We practically ignored Brent's four years of college because we were so overwhelmed with the governor's job. In one way, it forced him to grow up fast, I guess, and in another way, he was deprived of his parents. He missed some parenting during those early years, too. It didn't seem to hurt him, particularly, as he's a fine young man.

Looking back, maybe I should have kept Brent out a year; he started school at five and was the youngest child in his class. Both of my boys grew up slowly, and they didn't go through puberty until they were fifteen. Brent grew two inches just after he went away to college, and he gained about twenty pounds, which was good because he had been a skinny boy. My grandsons are the same way.

But Brent's done well; he is very successful. Recently, he sold his Little Rock cookie company for millions of dollars. The cookies were called Brent and Sam's, and the Giant grocery store and Whole Foods carried them. Whole Foods was competing nationally, and Brent baked their Nature's Promise brand of cookies. The cookie company was a real entrepreneurial effort. Brent started baking cookies while he was still in college. He tried different recipes and would put the cookies in little bags and have his friends test them until he perfected the recipes. He wanted to make the best chocolate chip cookie ever. Brent is really a good businessman with a gourmet palate. He knew what tasted good, and he put in big chunks of pecans and Ghiradelli chocolate and other good products. He didn't buy seconds or add just little bits—Brent knew how to keep a gourmet cookie a gourmet cookie. He said, "I'm Babe Flanagan if he'd had an education." And I guess that is true, as he has done very well.

I got the lesson of honesty from my mother, my dad, and my grandparents. It was just one of those important lessons, being honest. I got caught in a terrible lie one time. I really don't remember all of the details, but I just remember sobbing in my bed and my dad kind of consoling me. He just pressed on so hard for the truth that I finally fessed up to telling a lie. I don't even remember what it was about, but I remember the lesson: It doesn't pay to lie. So I have tried to not to lie or to cheat people.

Dale is a purist, given the way he was raised. I decided early on that was a wonderful way to raise children. You raise them with black-and-white rules until they reach the age of discretion. Then you begin to tell them when not to say to somebody, "You're ugly." You try to teach them to be discreet. And I tried to help them learn that you don't say, after a certain age, things like, "No, I don't like that, it is ugly." Or if someone asks, "Am I pretty?," you don't say, "No." You don't lie, but you find something beautiful about them to talk about. You say, "Yeah, you've got pretty hands," or, "Your eyes are so beautiful, of course you're not ugly."

Kids live by example. If you, as the parent, don't live that way, you don't hide one nuance from children. They pick up on anything and everything. In the meantime, you have to add on the layers of teaching. I'm working on this with one of my little grandchildren now, and I had to do it with one of my sons. My son had this famous imagination, and he would be in the backyard playing and come running into the house totally out of breath and say, "Oh, a lion was after me, mother. A lion was chasing me. He was out there by the storm cellar. He jumped up on the other side of that storm cellar and chased me all the way home." His eyes would be this big, and I would just try to calm him down.

I'd say, "We aren't going to pay any attention to you if you make things up." He would come in and tell us something, and we would say, "Well, we don't really know whether to believe you or not." It took me three years to teach him the difference between imagination or fantasy and telling a lie. I said, "Imagination has good things about it, and yours is wonderful. Maybe someday you will write fantastic stories. But you've got to learn how to separate all of that. And telling lies is connected to being dependable because if you lie, nobody can ever depend on you for anything."

My kids also used to exaggerate. They would come in and say, "Why can't we have a motorbike? All of our friends have motorbikes." And I would say, "Well, they may have a motorbike, but they won't go to college, and you will." Or it would be, "All of our friends have a car," and I'd say, "You can't have a car until you are old enough to drive and pass your driver's license. Then we will let you have the car as often as we can spare it. But no, we are not buying you a car when you get to be sixteen."

They'd say, "Well, so and so has one." And I'd say, "Well, they aren't going to college, but you are. We can't afford to both buy a car and save money to send you to college." When they kept asking for something their friends had, I sometimes said, "Some people spit on the floor, but we don't." Finally, it got to the point where they would come in and say, in a whiny voice, "Why can't we ———?" I would open my mouth, and they would say, "We know, we know."

I teach from my experiences. That time I panicked when I was new at the Fort Smith junior high, I realized that all you need to do is ask someone. Children need to learn that. Don't panic, ask! I have used that so many times with my children and my grandchildren. I say, "If you ever get bitten by a snake or if you ever have a horrible cut or an accident or other emergency—don't act like a chicken with its head cut off."

You know how those chickens will act. I used to be the one assigned to wring the fryers' heads off because I had learned how to do that snap. And chickens flop around and jump. I used to feel so terrible about the chicken jumping after its head was off, and my mother used to say, "Well, that's good because it pumps all the blood out." Then she would cut the chicken up and put it in saltwater to draw out the rest of the blood. And knowing that, I used to say, "Don't act like a chicken with its head cut off. Sit down and call for help. Because if you jump back like a chicken with his head off when you're cut, all your blood pumps out of your body. Or if you are bitten by a snake, you stir up the circulation, and that venom goes through your system faster. So what you need to do is sit down calmly and call for help." I just related all these things to that experience of the first day of middle school, and everybody does that; that is not unique.

Being the First Lady of Arkansas was such a learning experience for me. I do have the ability to be a good observer, to integrate all of the things I have learned and try to use them. I found out early that you use every experience you've had sometime later in your life, whether it is a bad experience, a good experience, or a mediocre experience. Growing up on a farm has been extremely valuable to me, even the tough stuff, like learning how to milk a cow when I was five and being happy to have the responsibility to do a good job with that. Other experiences, like having to travel in a truck taking care of calves, pay off sooner or later in your life.

I started understanding this after putting my foot in my mouth with the immunization campaign. When I'd said that Arkansas people don't need any more education, they just need to get the children immunized, I was trying to defend us against a hillbilly image. I had no idea, no concept, of how we would do that. Then I had to sit down and figure out how I was going to do it. So I just looked back and called on the things I had learned following my dad around behind a plow, about the Agricultural Extension people, and going to the canning kitchens with my mother as a little girl. I thought about what I'd learned as a schoolteacher and as a young adult going away to college and then coming back. When I went out of state, Iowa State was already fully integrated, and that was the first time I had been in a classroom with or sat next to or ate with black people. I realized they are just people; they are my friends. It was like what I realized later about the Soviet women I met later when Dale was a senator and we traveled to the USSR. They were mothers and fathers who wanted futures for their families.

So when I was figuring out how to immunize Arkansas children, I thought about the experiences I'd had and asked, why not use some of those old organizations? That was the genius of using in-place organizations and agencies and tapping into their agendas. I also knew that my husband appointed the heads of those departments, so when I went to them as the governor's wife, they jumped through hoops to please me, to cooperate and work with me. I tried not to lord that over them, but just to be aware that was a fact of life and that I was doing it for the children's immunizations.

If I had any talent, it was that ability to see and relate to the different needs that I had experience with. I could figure out how to solve needs, how to take care of them. A lot of people could do the same thing—teach school or help the PTA as health officer or organize volunteers—without becoming aware of what the real needs are. It is kind of a visionary thing, but if I have any real talent, that's probably it. I had to have the experience of a small town, of teaching in the school, to realize what the needs are. And I had to pay attention to those needs and be aware of them.

CONNECTIONS

BETTY BUMPERS AND HER INFLUENCE ON ARKANSAS

PAULA AGEE

"Betty Bumpers was the forerunner of the modern Governor's mate. Her tenure was pivotal for the first ladies of this state: Improving the quality of life for people in her state and later her country and the world," claims her longtime friend and Dale Bumpers's office manager, Linda Miesner.[1]

In longtime Arkansas journalist Ernie Dumas's documentary transcripts, Dale Bumpers recalls that "the first year I was governor; mostly she [Betty] spent her time on social things at the mansion, which she deplored frankly. She didn't enjoy that. She wanted to do something meaningful, particularly with children."[2]

As First Lady of Arkansas, "She wanted to do something that meant something: Something for Arkansas. She was looking for things that would be a contribution," her nephew Archie Schaffer said.[3] Her friends, Jean Gordon and Dr. Pat Youngdahl, agreed and added that she was not personally ambitious. "She didn't do things for show."[4] Without exception, her friends and family admire her work, but maybe more important, dozens of Arkansans who did not know Betty Bumpers personally have great respect for Mrs. Bumpers and her contribution to this state, primarily her efforts with immunization.

One of the people Betty went to for advice about the immunization program was Dr. Roger Bost,[5] friend and pediatrician for the Bumpers's children, as well as the director of health and human services during Governor Bumpers's tenure. Dr. Bost had practiced in Arkansas, and he saw firsthand the needs in the state. He remembers when there was an absence of health care, physicians, and hospitals: a great need in the state for acute care and long-term care for physical illness as well as a great need for those with mental and physical disabilities. Many counties relied on public health nurses as their only health care provider.

Archie Schaffer notes that for a long time he got "lots of comments about the impact" of the immunization drive and subsequent laws for which Betty worked. "All through the 1970s and 1980, it was a topic of great contribution to the children of the state at the time. And now, we see the next generation of children who have enjoyed the benefits of immunization and are looking at their children's children, and hopefully they are educated about the benefits of immunization for children."[6] Katheryn Bost hopes that future generations will remember Betty for her outstanding "stance on health." For a poor state like Arkansas with limited health care in the 1970s, immunization programs, initiated through Betty Bumpers's work, had a huge impact on the health and economics for people of this state.[7]

Betty's training and experience as an educator and a scholar prepared her for life: for decisions, for new experiences, for expression of who she would be as a member of this society. "While diverse in her interests and activities, she never lost the base of education," says nephew Archie Schaffer. "As an educator, she knew how to reach the audience. Probably someone else could have done it, but she was the right person to do it because she had the bully pulpit as the First Lady of the state and the passion to get it done and the educational 'how to do it' to get it done."[8] Betty Bumpers raised the bar for First Ladies of Arkansas.

Ernie Dumas observes, "I don't think that Betty thought a minute about Dale's politics. She doesn't appear to. He was upset about every little thing that came along. He was very impatient and reactionary. She was the calm one."[9] In Dumas's transcripts, Dale is quoted, "And Betty said, 'Why do you worry about junk?' Her words were, 'Why do you worry about crap like that?'"[10] She never worried about what she said when she thought it needed to be said or [worried about] its affecting Dale's political career. "It probably never hurt him, in fact [it] may have gained him respect, but it added some kind of mystique. Dale was always doing what he thought was right whether it was popular or not, and you respected him for it. She kept her husband thinking and standing up for 'what you know is right and don't worry about what the press or people say.' She helped shape that. [It] may be one of the most important contributions [of Betty Bumpers to our state]," notes Dumas.[11]

Linda Miesner agreed with Dumas's observation but tempered it slightly: "It was a great contribution but not her greatest. She did keep Dale in check and grounded and calm. He worried about it, but he worried about it less because of Betty."

"Betty was always Betty." Linda Miesner continued, "If Betty likes you, she likes you. She accepts people as individuals. She is opinionated, but she would never be unkind or ungracious. She doesn't suffer fools gladly regardless of your station, your power, your pedigree, or the color of your skin."[12]

William Sonny Walker, the first African American cabinet member appointed in 1968 by Governor Rockefeller, believes that "Dale would not have been the governor he was without Betty as his best friend and supporter." Sonny Walker gives a lot of credit to Betty and how she elevated the African American community. He was "impressed with her style and class and teased Dale Bumpers about 'marrying-up.' She was always comfortable with others. She came across as real, not artificial. She reached out across all kinds of lines. Betty touched people across racial lines, socioeconomic lines, and educational lines."[13] She treated everyone with respect and dignity and influenced those around her to do the same.

Prior to becoming Arkansas's First Lady, Betty was teaching fourth grade, and Dale served as the Charleston School District's attorney when it was the first of only two districts (the second was Fayetteville, Arkansas), not only in the state but also in the South, to integrate in 1954. Betty Bumpers was raised with a tolerance of other races, other socioeconomic statuses. Later, Betty was teaching Sunday school, and Dale was directing the choir and sat on the church board when their home church, First Methodist Church, Charleston, invited their sister African American Methodist church to join their congregation. Though they had supported the sister church over the years, Dale expressed in Dumas's transcripts that "they were so proud of themselves that we had integrated that church, which is the exemplification of Christianity. Everybody was tickled to death about it."[14]

More than her speech, Betty Bumpers's reputation and her ability to maintain long-term friendships across the state afforded her a receptive audience for her causes, including Peace Links. Using the model from her immunization drive, her passion for peace inspired women throughout the state. The participants were as committed to Betty as they were to the pursuit of peace. Youngdahl and Gordon agreed that "they related to her because of shared experience as mothers and sisters but also admired her for her privilege as a senator's wife."[15] Betty's unusual ability to be as down to earth as a neighbor and as enlightened as a world leader made her message palatable as well as igniting.

Jean Gordon, who served as chair of Peace Links after Sarah Murphy, shared that she attended the first big public meeting for what would become Peace Links wearing a button that said something like "Resist Authority," and Betty said, "Take that button off!" She was not having any of that, so Jean took the button off. Some folks think Betty soft-pedaled it. Jean agreed and admitted she would have said that. It was not Betty's style to protest, but she was also very intentional about presenting a credible message. Mrs. Gordon adds, "It takes courage to step out. She knew she was not the best speaker in the whole world. She didn't like it much. She didn't like it at all. She was doing things that were not easy for her—stepping out of her comfort zone. That is one thing I really admire her for because it is not easy to be up for ridicule for making a mistake. The papers can misquote you. She stretched and did it anyway."[16]

Roger Bost wants his grandchildren to remember "the kind of person she stood for. How she conducted herself. How she lived. How she related to other people, by virtue of who she was, what she believed, what she stood for, what she was capable of. What adjectives? Generous, down to earth, caring, concerned, outspoken, practical, wasn't afraid of anything, brave."[17]

While there was little lasting criticism of Betty Bumpers or her causes, Ernie Dumas remembers a certain out-of-state newspaperman who editorialized that "all this inoculation is not about helping kids but about getting Dale elected to the Senate."[18] While it is true that the publicity of Every Child by '74 was abundant and though most folks thought that

Betty's work helped her husband's career, this cynical criticism did not rally a lot of support.

Ernie Dumas surmises that "even those who have been put off by her respected her."[19] A strong feminist might say Betty rode on her husband's coattails. While she was not an early women's rights advocate, Betty's father's confidence in her abilities "always made her feel equal," and her feminist interests evolved over time.[20] Youngdahl observed, "In the early days of the women's movement, there were studies that showed that the women who had support from their fathers—the women whose fathers said you are still feminine and you are still a woman but you can do this—those are the women who could lead. I didn't know Betty's folks, but I know Betty and her sister Ruth. Betty and Ruth both had permission to be strong women."[21]

Several women concur by drawing a distinction between being "Southern" and being what is affectionately called "hill people." Arkansas is a Southern state, and there are Southern women in our state, genteel Magnolias if you will. But Betty and others from Charleston distinguish themselves. Hill women have sturdiness about them—not in stature or build but tenacity. When somebody needs to pull the wagon, they are always there to "pull the wagon." Hill women did not enjoy the money, the affluence their Southern sisters enjoyed, so they adapted and persevered. They are strong. Hill people are friendly and neighborly but not nosey.

Linda Miesner speculates that "had she stayed in Charleston, she still would have been helping people—not in a condescending way but through education, the arts, reading programs, education for women." Betty was loved by her family, by the people of Charleston, by the people of the state of Arkansas. She was one of us."[22]

Sonny Walker sums it up: "Though Arkansas is the only Southern state that has not had a black representative in Congress, Arkansas has produced some positively progressive leadership, including Dale and Betty Bumpers. They had an impact because they were natives. Arkansas is better off because of Dale and Betty Bumpers. Arkansas is better off for having Betty Bumpers as First Lady."[23]

Miesner's assessment of Betty Bumpers includes that "[her] lasting impact will be a First Lady who was very strong willed and independent but had a great deal of concern and felt a responsibility, a duty, to do the best she could for the state of Arkansas and for the people of Arkansas. Betty is not a complicated woman with lots of secret ambitions or desires. She was not a prima donna or a talking head. She was not threatening although as a First Lady, she had opinions, with issues, concerns, causes, missions."[24]

Betty's father, Babe Flanagan, was a farmer, a cattleman from whom Betty inherited a few hundred acres of virgin prairie. It has never been plowed and worked. Conservation is important to Betty. She has an interest in saving the land in its purest form. So Betty donated the land to The Nature Conservancy in Arkansas and named it Flanagan's Prairie. Miesner notes that it is "a lovely gift to the state to preserve land for wildlife and study." Betty's faith calls her to be a good steward in all things.[25] "When Betty would come to visit [the homestead in Charleston], she would be in the garden," recalls nephew Archie Schaffer.[26]

Arkansas senator David Pryor is quoted, "Betty Bumpers has had more impact than most on causes that are noble and good—and even holy—in our state and the nation."[27] According to Ernie Dumas, "[Dale] Bumpers reflects, 'She was a much more important person than I ever was.'"

NOTES

1. Linda Miesner (Bumpers's governor's mansion manager and friend), telephone interview by Paula Agee, November 28, 2010.
2. Dale Bumpers, interview by Ernie Dumas (from his personal notes and transcripts), for Arkansas Governors Project, University of Arkansas Little Rock, May 12, 2002.
3. Archie Schaffer (Bumpers's nephew), interview by Paula Agee, May 10, 2010.
4. Dr. Pat Youngdahl and Jean Gordon (Bumpers's friends), interview by Paula Agee, May 19, 2010.
5. Dr. Roger Bost and Katheryn Bost (Bumpers's pediatrician and friends), interview by Paula Agee, May 19, 2010.
6. Schaffer, interview.
7. Katheryn Bost, Bost and Bost interview.
8. Schaffer, interview.
9. Ernie Dumas, interview by Paula Agee, May 19, 2010.
10. Dale Bumpers, Dumas interview.
11. Dumas, interview.
12. Miesner, interview.
13. Sonny Walker, interview by Paula Agee, May 15, 2010.
14. Dale Bumpers, Dumas interview.
15. Youngdahl and Gordon, interview.
16. Gordon, Youngdahl and Gordon interview.
17. Roger Bost, Bost and Bost interview.
18. Dumas, interview.
19. Dumas, interview.
20. Betty Bumpers, Betty Bumpers and Joan Baker interview by Paula Agee, May 19, 2010.
21. Youngdahl, Youngdahl and Gordon interview.
22. Miesner, interview.
23. Walker, interview.
24. Miesner, interview.
25. Miesner, interview.
26. Schaffer, interview.
27. Paula Barnes, "Betty Flanagan Bumpers: 'An Ordinary Mother' Dedicated to Peace," in *Ordinary Women, Extraordinary Lives: Women in American History*, ed. Kriste Lindenmeyer (Wilmington, DE: Scholarly Resources, 2000), 248.

EIGHT

Living on the D.C. Beltway

Having been a governor's wife and then a Senate wife, I used who I was shamelessly. With those roles, I called on people to do things, and they responded because of my visibility. Not to diminish who I was because it took my tenacity and my willingness to see it through.

CONVERSATIONS WITH BETTY

I did not do a lot for Dale's first Senate campaign because he was such a popular governor. He beat Bill Fulbright in the primaries, and in the general election, he didn't have to do a lot of campaigning against the other candidate, John H. Jones, a man from the Clark candy family, who ran a token campaign against him. So the only race where Dale faced real opposition was that first run for governor. Though I didn't need to do much for the first Senate campaign, I went out when he ran for his second term. Brooke was old enough for that, so she and I started going around to the courthouses and shaking hands.

After that governor's race, when my sisters, Bequita, and I had done a lot of campaigning, people thought they already knew me. After we did that door-to-door knocking in so many towns in southeastern and southwestern Arkansas and around Fort Smith, for years everybody thought that we had come to see them personally, that I had knocked on their doors. I have heard so many stories blown out of proportion about my knocking on their doors and the conversations we've had. It has always been very amusing and heartwarming.

I was so involved in my own issues by that time that I didn't come home to Arkansas very often. But the people didn't really miss me because Dale talked about me a lot, and they thought that I played a role in his campaign because he described what I was doing. Of course, I was also well known from when we had immunized so many kids on one Saturday in 1973.

During Dale's Senate races, Brooke agreed to go with me and talk about overall issues. She was in college by this time and more attuned with them. I was on top of peace and conflict issues because I was so involved with Peace Links, the network I had started to activate women against the threat of nuclear war. Brooke kept up more with the specific issues that Dale dealt with in the Senate, and she agreed to make brief speeches at courthouses. In Arkansas, the courthouses are built in the town squares. The stores and shops surround the squares, and the politicians meet and hold rallies right out there. They use the beds of trucks as speaking platforms. We went to the towns and just started walking around the courthouses, where all the people would be milling about, waiting for the political speakers to show up. I would shake hands and introduce myself to people, talk to them, chitchat with them.

At one courthouse where I handed out literature with Brooke, I got halfway around and said, "Brooke, where are you?" I had noticed Brooke kept lagging behind me, and she was not handing out literature. Finally, she said, "I don't mind getting on the back of that truck and making a little speech, but this one-on-one crap is not for me." So she quit doing that and wouldn't even get out of the car until it was time for her to stand up and give her talk.

Another reason I didn't work on the first Senate campaign was because I was so involved with immunization; I continued that work during Dale's first six years in the Senate. Jimmy Carter was elected president two years after Dale came to the Senate, and he had made immunization an issue in his campaign. Even though Carter was later defeated for reelection, I stayed involved in the state-by-state immunization work with Rosalynn Carter. I began looking at Peace Links because Brooke was growing up and still in high school, and I organized it and we got it started by 1982 (see chapter 3).

When Dale was governor, we went to Washington, D.C., for the National Governors Association conference. When the group meets there, it has a dinner at the White House, and for our first dinner there, I sat at the table with President Richard Nixon. Dale had been running in the Democratic primary against Bill Fulbright, chair of the Senate Foreign Relations Committee and a powerful figure in Washington.

Bill was not campaigning well—it was one of those cases of not coming back to the state often or paying enough attention to the state, and Dale was a very popular governor. He outcampaigned Bill and beat him soundly in the primary, too, later that spring. Dale was doing well in his Senate campaign, and he was looking like the golden boy of the day, so I sat at the president's table. I went downtown and bought this beautiful gown—going to the White House, oh my! It was pale yellow and pink with beading on it, a gorgeous dress and matching coat for being seated next to Nixon. Later, I gave the outfit to the Old State House Museum of History, and it is on display in Little Rock.

When they brought out the finger bowls, each had this lacey leaf and a white geranium blossom. The leaves were very scented, and with it smelling like geranium, I really didn't know what to do with that finger bowl. Nixon sort of picked up on it, and I just watched and followed suit. I had mentioned the beautiful leaf, and he said, "You know, Mrs. Bumpers, that leaf came from plants on the top of the White House. They grow up there and are stripped to be used for precisely this." I just went on about the scented water, and he called the waiter over. The waiter was Rex Sutton, who recently retired after being there for thirty or forty years. Nixon said, "Send this young lady a plant." So Nixon sent me a scented geranium; he was charming and delightful.

I had called on Pat Nixon when I was working on immunizations and met with her about volunteers, and she helped me out. She was a doer and more personable than most people thought. She wasn't all that wimpy; controlled was what she was, in a lot of ways, and by him, I suppose. But she was a nice woman who had moxie. I enjoyed the little contact I had with her. I remember the night so well when he sent me that plant because it was his last year. When we came to Washington in January 1975, he had left office the previous summer, 1974. The Watergate investigations were taking place all of this time, and the call was for his resignation.

Then Gerald Ford came in, and Betty Ford struck me as a rather sad figure. She, of course, had breast cancer, but even before that she seemed depressed. She was a sweet, low-key person, and I was around her several times, but I didn't know her very well. Later, she set up the Betty Ford Center.

Then there were the Carters, and I've already said so much about the immunization and how Rosalynn and Jimmy helped (see chapter 2). After them, the Reagans. Ronald Reagan had served his last two years as governor of California while Dale was still governor. I knew Nancy from that time when we were both state First Ladies, but of course I also had known of her when I worked at Passavant Hospital in Chicago. Her mother, Mrs. Davis, was head of the hospital auxiliary and worked in the café, and she was one of the women who hired me to work in the library. Dr. Davis was the top neurosurgeon in the country. He was Nancy's stepfather, but I think he had raised her. Sometimes Dr. Davis would do brain operations lasting eight hours or longer, and he would come to the library and meet Mrs. Davis. He would just take a break there or at the café and get off of his feet. So I knew both of her parents and had heard about Nancy.

The first governors' conference we went to after Dale was elected was in Puerto Rico. I was out on the beach one day and noticed two or three state police standing around. I looked over, and there were Governor and

First Lady Ronald and Nancy Reagan, in matching brown and white polka-dot bathing suits. I thought I'd go over and ask about her father and mother because it had been fifteen or sixteen years since I had worked with them. When I walked over, the police tried to stop me, and I had to tell them who I was. The Reagans kind of looked up at me, and I introduced myself and asked about her parents.

Nancy said, "Father is a semi-invalid, and they are living in Sun City; they are doing very well, thank you." And with that I was dismissed. You know, she just let me know I was interrupting their time together. So I left, but it always kind of smarted. She never recognized me again or connected that exchange to anything about her mother or Chicago; she never knew who I was from a load of hay.

The year that Reagan was elected president, four or five governors were elected to either the Senate or Congress. Every year, the wives of the senators have a luncheon for the First Lady, and then she reciprocates. The Senate ladies' luncheon is held in different places, like at the botanical gardens, but most of the time it is in the caucus room of the Russell Senate Office Building, a beautiful place overlooking Constitution Avenue. That year, we had our luncheon, and Nancy Reagan reciprocated in May and had all the Senate ladies to the White House. She did not have the congressional wives there because there were too many of them. In the receiving line, she did not recognize but one of the governors' wives, who'd been state First Ladies when she was. She knew Governor Williams's wife from Arizona, and that was because her mother and father lived in an assisted-living facility in that state. She didn't even recognize me, though we had sat with each other at many governors' events at least briefly.

The Reagans never stayed long for any event. Nancy was not good with crowds, and I attributed it to her being a shy actress. I never did care about her causes, the "Just Say No" stuff that she subscribed to. Some of the issues she took on were good, but some were not significant as far as I was concerned.

The Senate wives still have lunch with the First Lady every year, and I try to go to most of the luncheons to see old friends. It is fun to see the White House, and it is always a great reunion, as the wives are invited even after their husbands are out of office.

A lot of the Senate wives helped with Peace Links. I had over 170 congressional or Senate wives, though a lot of them only lent their names because their husbands wouldn't let them be involved with such a "commie" thing. They were afraid it might affect their reelection or people would hear about it back in their voting districts. But most wives just didn't do any volunteering or work on projects. Now the Senate has a lot of working wives, many of whom are attorneys, and it is a very different scene than when I was first there. A lot of Senate wives are significant women in their own right, but none of them have taken on something so controversial or daring as Peace Links. Of course, I didn't realize that what I was doing was that different.

We attended some of the inaugurations, including Jimmy Carter's and Bill Clinton's. Sometimes during those years we took part in that sort of historical occasions, and we had some other interesting experiences. Dale and I flew on Air Force One with the Clintons when Bill was president. A good mutual friend, Diane Kincaid Blair, had died back in Arkansas. Diane was a political science professor at the University of Arkansas who worked with Bill's campaign, and she was a close friend of Hillary. Bill and Hillary invited us to fly with them to Diane's funeral, which was very considerate, and it was neat being on Air Force One.

Hillary was and is still so popular internationally, among women in China and India and Africa. Outside of women in this country, others see her as a powerful leader. Besides that, she and Bill changed the attitudes about daughters just by the way they treated Chelsea. Chelsea was always standing by them in photos, and there were lots of pictures of her with President Clinton, and she traveled with him some. Bill and Hillary valued her and raised the status of women in a lot of countries. People loved Hillary and Chelsea. I don't think the world knows how much.

I still hear occasionally from a lot of friends that I made in Russia. Dr. Billington, who headed up the delegation from the Senate when I first went there, was a Russian teacher and expert. We traveled there just after Reagan had called the Soviets "the evil empire." Senator Byrd recruited eight Democratic senators and their wives to take a junket, which is what they call the Senate trips. We went to Russia to convey to the Russians that there was another attitude in this country besides the evil empire attitude. We had a very extensive, wonderful trip. We went to Moscow and to Leningrad before they called it St. Petersburg. From there we went down to Samarkand, to Georgia, to Tashkent. That was when I realized that the Russian people were the victims of the same thing that we were. The women just hadn't had any leadership. Instead of them being called a communist for peace work, they'd be punished, and it was a danger to their whole family, too. I made lots of contacts on that trip

Thank God for this wonderful interpreter that we had on that first trip. You know how sometimes you meet people and you just have instant friendship, bonding? Well, she and I did. She taught at a university, but she had offered to go on this trip as an interpreter just to get to travel. She had never been out of Moscow, except once the Soviet government sent her to England, as they did a lot of teachers, to learn English.

Every time Dale got up out of his seat on the plane, flying from here to there, my interpreter friend came and sat down with me. So we just had such a great bonding, and she made herself available at banquets and meetings where most Senate wives just sat there with their husbands. I was interested in talking to other women, so my interpreter arranged for me to meet with some of the Soviet wives and other women just out in the lobby of places where we were. She understood my curiosity. At that time I was beginning to question a lot of things even before I started Peace Links. I found out, during that time, you didn't dare ask these Soviet women if they were communists or if they were Christians or anything like that. But our interpreter let me know because she took me to an ancient church. She asked if I wanted to light a candle. I didn't know where to go get the candle to light, and I said, "Well, if you want to."

She said, "I've already lit mine." That was her way of telling me that she was a believer, that she was not a communist.

When I talked to Soviet women, I would just ask them how they felt about the arms race, the security of their country, the future. And they would talk to me. They were just as open as American women. I found that they felt comfortable with our interpreter. I'm sure she had a lot to do with their openness with me.

She was very open about their bomb shelters and everyday security. My God, their bomb shelters were three feet underground. That's just as ridiculous as our government's civil defense direction for us to drive out of Washington in case of a nuclear blast. How the hell were we going to get out of Washington on that two-lane highway in time with millions of people driving? The Soviet women felt the same way. I would just ask them questions that were simple enough that they understood, and that's when it solidified in my head that they really felt the same way we did.

Then later in Peace Links, we thought of the Soviet women's visit because when I would travel around our country, I was talking about how outraged I was and what was happening to us. It also happened to the Soviet people, and they felt the same way as we did. But then so many American people would say, "We feel so and so, but how about the Russians?" I thought, well, there's no reason why we can't let them come speak for themselves because I had talked to so many of them.

My first interpreter was not a member of the Soviet Women's Committee, but I met some of them through Collette Shulman, newspaper reporter and a Soviet Union contact, and Debbie Harding, who helped me start Peace Links. Debbie and I went to New York to the Soviet Mission. Through that Soviet Mission and Collette Shulman, the next time I made a trip to Moscow I met with the Soviet Women's Committee at their headquarters. Most of them were not communists. It was the only women's network left in Russia, the only one that was allowed to flourish. Of course, they had to use Russian philosophy and all, but many of them were not communist as it turns out.

When I went to meet the Soviet Women's Committee, I remember trying to cross that square in Moscow from my hotel. This main street runs through the big circle where all the roads meet, with about twelve lanes across it. I remember being so dumb I didn't know that they had the underground passage. I finally made it across the square but only because they had so few cars.

At the Soviet Women's Committee headquarters, I went in and sat down in this little room with these fancy chairs, and they had their interpreter. I remember sitting and talking to the president and two head honchos and asking them questions. They talked to me because I was so candid with them. For one thing I said, "Are you women in the Soviet Union like the women in America, dumped on with everything from working to doing all the housework? Are you burdened with either sticking something up or down yourself for birth control or going through abortions?"

They'd punch each other, and they just could not believe that somebody would talk to them so candidly. So I was an instant star and a hit. They would answer my questions. Oh they loved it. Of course, they had no birth control, so they just went through seven or eight abortions in their lives, without anesthetic most of the time. The most frequent thing I took as gifts on all the trips that I made back and forth to Russia was a suitcase full of condoms. I said if I had ever been stopped and opened that suitcase, and here I have a suitcase full of condoms, what would they do? I couldn't get a big enough bunch of [birth control] pills. I just remember making that gift, and word spread through their organization. So I was always welcomed with open arms by every Soviet Women's Committee in the many cities I went to. The committee got out the word, even though they're nine time zones away from each other. Those women had plenty of money and were very well connected; they'd travel back and forth. Valentina Tereshkov, the first woman astronaut, was a member of it; so was Gorbachev's wife, Riesa.

Later I did a television program with Riesa. I met her through Dr. Armand Hammer, a philanthropist who gave Peace Links a lot of money. I went to a big cultural meeting that he convened. He was presenting Mrs. Gorbachev with around twenty old Russian master paintings that he had collected over all the years. I went to the Museum of Art with him and Mrs. Hammer, and Riesa met us there. Riesa was accepting these paintings, and we both had on bright red dresses. I remember a few of my Soviet friends calling me at the hotel: "Poor Betty, we saw you and your beautiful red dress."

The Soviet women were not very supportive of Riesa Gorbachev. I thought she was smart, articulate, and well educated, as she accepted those paintings so graciously and commented on them. I had some of the worst disagreements with Soviet Women's Committee, even with my good friends there, who did not like her because she was just something brand new. Progress comes in tiny increments. Some women just could not make that transition from that old traditional role where a wife never made an appearance. They just thought Riesa was an uppity woman. Even the most progressive Russian women did not like her. Now they feel pretty bad. I've heard several of them express themselves: "We just didn't understand. She was too modern."

Up until recently, I volunteered with peace organizations. Senators Matsunaga, Hatfield, and Jennings Randolph dreamed up that National Peace Academy, and the idea spread fast. The National Peace Foundation was the grassroots support that kept alive the dream of a National Peace Academy. Those senators came up with legislation that created the national U.S. Institute of Peace. They finally got it through Congress. For a while, I was on the U.S. Institute of Peace board. Their leadership has been uneven, but they do very good things in teaching conflict resolution. When I joined their board, they did not have a congressional liaison, and I fought to get that started. You may not realize how important that is, but it's how things work in Washington—through who you know and through the Congress. Congress appropriates the money and passes the laws. So I said, "Get a congressional liaison with a couple of staff members and start putting your positions out there. I can't tell you how those senators and congressmen are looking for talking points, especially when they go back to their home states. Because problems arise, and they would love to say, 'Oh, in this conflict, the U.S. Institute of Peace has come to this conclusion: that we should do so and so and so.' They would love to have a one-pager on something like that."

Institute leaders don't have enough imagination about that. I said, "Ninety-nine percent of the senators up there, including my husband, who voted to form this organization aren't even aware that you exist." That's true. So now they have a congressional liaison, but they still don't connect enough to Congress. They have a very good person as chair of the board who is a Republican and understands that. And he is always chiding me, "Well, if you want to know where Betty stands just ask. You don't even need to ask her, we all know."

The institute could be a more vital resource, although I give them credit for several things. They did a lot of the groundwork and the solution in Bosnia. They are doing a lot of conflict resolution training in Iraq and Darfur. They have a lot of real experts out there trying to teach conflict resolution, but they could be engaging so many more educational institutions in this country about the fact that we have a U.S. Institute of Peace. People could turn to the institute. It is just one of those things, it will take time. I am impatient. I think things ought to move faster than they do.

I did what I did in Peace Links because I was competitive, and I wanted to make a mark in ending the arms race. I just let people know, "Stop and think about what we allow. We, the American people, allowed this to happen." It's happening right now. Ordinary people allowed the military planners to build all of those nuclear weapons when we knew we could never dare use them. What was wrong with Americans? What is still wrong with us that we allow stupid planners to do this? Think what we could be doing in this country. The infrastructure is crumbling down because we don't have money. We don't have money for public schools; it's so pitiful. Yet we allow them to spend billions on weapons and wars. How much have the Iraq and Afghanistan wars cost us so far? It is sad, but we've gone through this all through history, and here we go again. The point is that once again we need strong leadership for the peace movement, just like we did with Peace Links. People need to stop being intimidated, to stand up and talk about it.

Dale and I have participated in historical events during that time in Washington. We had some good times and some challenges and illnesses. I've mentioned my tenacity as a reason I succeeded with the immunization programs and with Peace Links. And I think that is one reason I survived these illnesses: I just refused to give up.

Around the time I was getting interested in Peace Links, I had to have surgery. I explained that to the doctor when I went in for a colon resection. He said, "Is there anything you want to say or that we need to talk about before surgery?"

I explained to him about what I did and didn't want done for me during the surgery and recovery, and I said I didn't want pain medication unless I asked for it. When I told him I didn't want much pain medication, he tried an experiment with me. He was a top-class surgeon at Georgetown University, and he explained he had been trying a little device called a TENS unit. It has a small C battery that straps around the base, and it is placed on the incision. It causes a little vibration that can be dialed up and down.

I agreed to try it, and it did help with pain. After a nineteen-inch colon resection, I had only three pain shots and a couple of pain pills. It was my sister who talked me into taking the third shot. I had said, "I don't want any visitors, and I don't even want you to talk to me. I just want to lie still and get well." And so I did. I was back in Charleston two weeks and two days after the operation. I attended my mother's funeral, and I stood up straight.

My mother probably died of peritonitis from cancer treatments she had for several malignancies, but she was always clear of mind. Even in her late eighties, she was still up and walking around, though she was pretty debilitated. She was always a night person. When we were in Charleston, we'd pass by her house, and she would have the light on. She never went to bed before eleven or twelve o'clock; she would listen to the Chicago radio station that played music all night, or she would play card games. She didn't ever really get to bed for long and just sleep.

My mother died about six months before my dad. We had requested flowers and donations to the church or to the Cancer Society because my mother had beat five primary malignancies, and even at eighty-eight, she didn't die of cancer but its complications. But I remember writing thank-you notes to people who sent money to the church and saying that it had served five or six generations of my mother's family. I asked my dad about the actual number of generations, and we were trying to count back those that were either there in Charleston or nearby in Branch, where she grew up. He sat there for a few minutes, and because he knew at the time that he had lymphoma and that it was terminal, he said, "Well, Betty, when you do that for me, you can say the church served six generations of my family in Branch."

After Dale retired from the Senate in 1999, the one thing he missed was the companionship. He left because he just could not tolerate the caliber of people who were there anymore. It seemed they won their seats like they were in beauty contests on TV. Some of them are not well educated, and he feels that people almost have to have a legal education to understand the implications of laws and governing. At least we need a certain percentage of them who have legal educations and experience.

Some people in Congress now were TV personalities who read the news, and that's all. A lot of them are just, as he said, pretty boys who came across on TV wonderfully well. Others are millionaires, people who had enough money to be elected. They have almost no understanding of what they're doing. All they have in mind is being carried out of Congress in a box—and getting reelected until then.

Of course, Dale fought many unwinnable battles on the environment. He was the first one to talk about carbon cycle and about global warming, but they didn't listen. He was talking about the laws out West that allow mining companies to rape this country and leave us nothing but environmental problems to clean up. We don't even see any money from the dollar-an-acre leases that the mining companies get, and they haul out billions of dollars of coal and other valuable minerals.

Grazing lands are ruining our environment, but all that land is leased out to wealthy ranchers, rich people who don't care about whether they graze that grass too low and cause erosion. All of those were environmental problems—the mining and the grazing lands and the forests. Dale just got tired of losing all the battles for one thing. He had also developed a hearing problem. He just ran out of patience, so he didn't miss anything about the Senate except the camaraderie of his colleagues.

You know, usually men don't really have friends like women have or our network of support among women friends. They have acquaintances and colleagues but not friends. Dale went to work after he left the Senate, first at the Center for Defense Information for a year, but that turned out just to be a fund-raising position. He helped them get reorganized and on track, but fund-raising is not his cup of tea. He taught for a year, though he had taught previously only right after World War II. He didn't understand college kids, and he wondered why they didn't ask good questions at the end of his lectures or why they didn't know what questions to ask. He had expected them to be more sophisticated, and maybe he should have been teaching in graduate school instead of undergraduate. He was so disenchanted that he did not do it another year.

Dale ended up going into a law firm as an environmental lobbyist. One day he was complaining about having to eat lunch either by himself or with a colleague that he didn't enjoy much. I made a suggestion because he has so many ex-staff members here who are good friends and who love him, and he loves them, and he knows a lot of ex-senators and ex-congressmen who are lobbyists. I said, "Why don't you sit down and make a list of people you would like to have lunch with and just start inviting them?"

"Well, that's the best idea you've ever had," he told me. He really enjoyed that, and he had several clients, including one from Arkansas. He got a big national company as a client by picking up a man on his way to the Metro every morning at the ride-on stop. He had just stopped and picked somebody up, and this man was president of a large company that ended up as a client.

Dale's former staff members had a rotating routine for lunch, and he also enjoyed having lunch with seven or eight colleagues from the Senate. This reestablished that camaraderie. His colleagues greeted him like he was one of them, even though he didn't always vote with them a lot of times on certain issues. But he loved the work, and keeping in contact really helped him a lot.

Our family always tried to spend good time together. My daughters-in-law are very smart women, dear and wonderful people. LeAnn came from a small town in Oklahoma. After Brent got his undergraduate degree, he spent a lot of time with my sister Ruth, and she introduced him to LeAnn. Heidi is from California; she and Bill met while they both were working in environmental law. She was one of the women who started flextime in Washington, D.C., so that new mothers didn't start back to work until they had their children settled with care. Heidi created a flextime work schedule so that she could be home when her children got out of school.

When we lived in Washington, Brent's family came up from Arkansas to visit pretty often. And they celebrated special occasions. When I was inducted into the Women's Hall of Fame in 2005, Brent's wife, LeAnn, made sure that they all came to New York for the ceremony. She said, "I think it's time for our children to learn about their grandmother. I mean they're old enough now, and I'd love to have them come see their BB honored." The children knew all about Dale, but I wanted them to know about their "BB," too—the grandchildren call me "BB." They call Dale "Umpy" because one of the kids couldn't say grandpa. First it was "Umpa," and then they changed it to "Umpy" because it's easier to spell. Except for Brent, the rest of us lived close together in Bethesda. Brooke lived almost next door, with one house between us. Bill lived about a mile from us in a little suburb, an old community right off the river, and he practiced environmental law. His wife, Heidi, was still an environmental lawyer, too. We moved to Arkansas a few years after Dale retired from the Senate, when he retired from his other work in Washington.

Some call our politics "yellow dog Democrat," and that really indicates a philosophy: a belief in equality, in taking responsibility for helping other people, that we are our brother's keeper, that the rising tide lifts all of us. They believe in paying taxes and paying their fair share, even if, right now, some Republicans don't believe in that.

A lot of people don't like paying taxes, and they don't like helping the poor. They say, "Just pull yourself up by your own bootstraps." When they look at people who don't make it, they don't realize, as most Democrats say, "There but for grace of God go I." Of course, we Methodists grew up with some lessons from John Wesley, who founded the Methodist Church, and Susanna Wesley, his mother who is called the mother of the Methodist Church. The Wesleys' history was very democratic and very practical. God gave us a brain and turned us loose to use it, so Methodists don't stand by a lot of rules and regulations. The basic Sermon on the Mount and the Beatitudes had a lot to do with what we think.

CONNECTIONS

ROSALYNN CARTER[1]

From the very beginning, my support as First Lady was enlisted. Betty Bumpers, the wife of the former governor of Arkansas, Senator Dale Bumpers, and an old friend of mine, had been working on a childhood immunization program to eradicate measles . . . she came to me, not only as a friend, but because she knew I would bring it to the attention of Joe Califano, the secretary of the Department of Health, Education and Welfare. . . . I called him the same day and asked if he would talk with Betty, and Jimmy sent a note telling him to move forward on the program. During the next two years I helped them when called upon to generate publicity, or to get a wayward state in line, and the results were astounding. We reached our goal of immunizing 90 percent of the nation's children by October 1979 and have now, for all practical purposes, eliminated measles in the United States.

EXCERPTS FROM AN AUGUST 2005 INTERVIEW ON BETTY BUMPERS AND PEACE LINKS

CAROL WILLIAMS, DEMOCRATIC CAUCUS LEADER, MONTANA SENATE, FORMER PEACE LINKS EXECUTIVE DIRECTOR

The gift that Betty had was the vision and then the tenacity to go for the vision. There are a lot of tenacious people out there who don't get much done, but Betty would go on a trip out around the country and come back with this idea. "We've been doing things this way, and we can do this new idea." She could see how it would work out down the road, and a lot of people can't.

One of the good things that Betty came up with was the idea of getting congressional wives leadership programs to get them trained to go out and do the speeches she was doing. She'd just get a handful, three or four congressional wives, then bring somebody in to do a speaking training: How do you do it? How do you respond to questions? Here are some sample speeches, here's the data you need. Then send them off to their district to make a speech to the PTA. It was simple, dynamic, but people couldn't believe it actually worked.

The Peace Panel was kind of unique. We set it up partly to give Betty some help. The panel gave congressional wives new to the job the support of somebody else being there with them, someone from the audience or from the community who would join them. You had a group of different, new perspectives. It gave people who didn't want to get up and give a full-blown speech a comfort level. They could sit there and talk about their own little part of it.

It was so effective for the audience, too, because even if a good speaker gives a powerful keynote address, there's always another dimension to complicated things. If you have four people giving different perspectives, you have a much better chance to touch everybody in the audience because they all come to it differently with the ways they hear it or relate it to their own personal circumstances. The panel magnified our effectiveness to be able to do that plus gave Betty a little bit of a break from having to be the only one who was always pushed up there doing everything.

I wasn't sure this was going to work, but it worked great, and part of it worked because of Betty. She really made you feel empowered by the time that she picked you out of the audience. She would say things like, "I never used to like to speak, and it became such an important thing for me. I just go out and do it and my gosh. Sometimes it's not any good, and sometimes it's wonderful." We had people from all over writing to us saying, "You know I'm going to run to the school board or run for legislature." In the beginning, when the military started following us around, it was a little intimidating. There were a lot of women's organizations out there that were really nervous about having any antinuclear group as speakers, and so they'd invite the military to be a part of it. It had to be balanced. Normally we all hear the military side through all of our history, but, for our peace panels, we had to have somebody from the military there. We thought, you put one foot in front of the other, and we'll get to the end of it.

I could do the technical organizing but not the vision. I was so buried with the nitty-gritty that I didn't have the time or energy for the vision. But Betty always had the vision no matter how tired she got. She'd go out and travel, or she'd be ironing shirts. Suddenly, she'd say, "I was ironing shirts," and I would say, "Oh, shoot, she's got a new idea. I wonder how we'll fund this one."

It was always so hard to get money for Peace Links. In the early 1980s, we first got our big funding from the foundations. They had deep pockets, and they would fund peace organizations. In the 1980s we got funding when we were doing exchanges with the Soviet women. But basically foundations give you the money, and they expect you to go out and figure a way to sustain yourself. Well, it just isn't that easy, and then the foundation money dried up as soon as the Soviet Union started to go away; it would have been 1989, 1990. The Cold War was over, and people acted like there was not a threat anymore, so why do we do this? Betty always said they were like lemmings; someone in the foundation would start something and move forward. Everybody else would follow. They lost interest in peace, it wasn't sexy any more, and they moved on to other things.

When the Pen Pal project came along, that was another time of big growth; it wasn't financially very helpful. In fact, it was a big financial drain for a while. It began when we had a young woman intern who spoke Russian just write a letter to the Russian newspapers and say we're a group of American women who want to correspond with Russian women. Get in touch, and we'll find you a correspondent. We thought, "Nobody will print that. We'll never hear anything from that." And one day a guy down the street who monitored all the Russian newspapers called us: "Oh, by the way, your article's here," and we were shocked. In two weeks they were bringing mail to us, bags and bags. We said, "Now what do we do?" We had to go out and try to get national publicity so Americans would ask for pen pals, and it was huge for a while. We probably doubled the numbers of people who called themselves Peace Links from that project. So many people had never even thought of it because of the mystery of the Soviet Union.

During all of that, there were a lot of Senate wives out there, but they weren't doing what Betty was doing. When you think about how many young people came home to their mothers and did what Brooke did—wonder where their families would meet if there's a nuclear war. And their mothers didn't do anything except worry about it. Betty took it on because she had vision. Plus she was blessed to have gray hair and an

Arkansas accent. She could call someone a son of a bitch without them even knowing just because of the way she looked and sounded. I'm sure people thought she couldn't be threatening—look at her. The tenacity helped her keep on, but it was the vision that kept her going.

CONNECTIONS

KIND ACTS FROM BETTY

LARISA SKURATOVSKAYA (MOSCOW, RUSSIA)
TRANSLATED BY EDWARD VAJDA,
WESTERN WASHINGTON UNIVERSITY

I never imagined anyone would build bomb shelters in Moscow. . . . But today by chance I heard a broadcast of "Moscow Echo" that reported they were being built. Bomb shelters, now, in 2009, in Moscow? What for? The bomb shelter in the apartment building where we live on Leninskiy Prospect in the center of Moscow was long ago converted to a European-style restaurant in spite of determined resistance by the residents. This area also housed the building's entire communication network, and we did want it to be left undefended. . . . In Moscow many apartment buildings built from the 1930s to 1970s were equipped with bomb shelters. Judging from the number of restaurants and cafés situated in basements, all of the former bomb shelters have been refurbished for a more peaceful time. I again recalled these attributes of war, including the "cold" war, over the past few days as I was thinking what to write about Betty Bumpers, a faithful friend of our family and a brave woman—someone who helped put that "cold" and difficult war to rest. . . . Betty told how at the beginning of the 1980s she awoke once because her daughter was crying. When Betty asked her what had upset her, she said she was afraid that the Soviet Union would drop an atom bomb on Washington and she would die. At that time bomb shelters were being built all across America, and the press, radio, and television incessantly spoke both directly and indirectly of this as a real possibility. That happened several times despite the fact that Betty and Dale (who served as senator from Arkansas for a long time) kept explaining to their daughter that it wasn't going to happen. Betty talked to her friends, and it turned out that their families were also worried about this problem. Betty proposed to other senators' wives the idea of creating a nongovernmental organization, Peace Links—Women Against Nuclear War, as a way of somehow helping to diffuse this situation, which the professional politicians seemed to have driven into a troubling stalemate. Betty many times met with Soviet people, and she was convinced that they did not want war, just like other peoples of the world likewise didn't want war. Her idea caught on, and the nongovernmental organization was organized. When she met Valentina Vladimirovna Tereshkova, the first woman cosmonaut, who headed up the Committee of Soviet Women at that time, Betty passed on to her an invitation for fifteen women from the Soviet Union to visit America as guests of the newly created organization "in order to give Soviet people a human face," she said later. There was only one condition: The delegation should include not the same women who frequently traveled in delegations to the United States but instead other women from different layers of society. I am a doctor, and from the very inception of the international organization Physicians for the Prevention of Nuclear War, I have been an active member and still am. I had never traveled as a member of any delegation and was recommended as a member of this delegation by my friend, a wonderful woman and philosopher, Nelli Matroshilova, who was an active member of the committee. And so by pure chance I found myself a member of that unusual delegation, which indeed included members of all layers of society of the republics of our Soviet Union. I don't know how it is today, but at that time we would learn whether we had been given a visa only on the evening just before the departure date. That's how it happened this time, too. We all were very worried and not without reason. At the last moment it turned out that we weren't going to be traveling with Sveltana Askol'dova, a professor who had studied American history her entire career. She was sure that she had been turned down because of her husband, Aleksandr Askol'dov, whose film *The Commissar* had been banned and who had been subjected to all sorts of repressions though not openly. I felt sad that Sveta would not be traveling with us. After Washington, D.C., we were—the three of us from the delegation—supposed to travel to Utah, Arizona, and Nevada, states that the Soviet people had never visited and states that produced cutting-edge electronic technology as well as, unfortunately, atom bomb technology and nuclear weapons. . . .

I was incredibly, unbelievably fortunate since only a few days before our flight out of Moscow, our international movement, Physicians for the Prevention of Nuclear War, received the Nobel Peace Prize for 1985. . . . On that trip there were many wonderful meetings and coincidences. One of them was as follows. In the American delegation that was with us in Washington was Collette Shulman. She had worked for several years in the American embassy in Moscow, spoke Russian, and, I think, at that time was the best expert in Russia on the U.S. delegation. Collette spoke with the members of our delegation and with me as well. She delicately asked what I did, how I came to be in the delegation, where I lived in Moscow. . . . It turned out that she had been, since her embassy days, a friend of Marina Litvinova, who lived in the same apartment complex as I and was a friend of our family. This is how Collette and I happened to meet, and afterward she was a guest in our home a number of times. That trip gave me much new information. In the first place, I learned more about AIDS, an epidemic that was just getting under way. That gave me the opportunity to write a brief informative description for young people who came to the Youth Festival as a preventive measure. Afterward, I widely spread the word about means of prevention against this disease and invited a delegation from the United States that included doctors and relatives of AIDS patients as well as carriers of the virus. Through Clarita

Antonevska and Rosaline Lynch, activists in the antinuclear movement in Nevada, I met a wonderful woman doctor who is an obvious leader against the spread of nuclear energy and whose scientific and editorial articles gave such strong support to us all after the Chernobyl catastrophe in 1986. This was Rosalie Bertell, whose friendship greatly enriched me intellectually. For the first time I visited a hospice in Las Vegas. After returning home I also told people about this service to the seriously ill, which eases their farewell with this life. Later I met Victor Zorze, who came to Moscow to help open the first hospices in Moscow. How long ago all this was! When I talk about this wonderful trip, which influenced the rest of my life so significantly, and someone asks what year it took place in, there is always a pause after my answer. It seems long ago to them but not to me since I have maintained friendships with the people who traveled with me or who I met in America, and the name Betty Bumpers is a password to meeting new friends.

She changed a lot during that time, our Betty. . . . She became younger and more attractive. She cut her hair and used a bit of lipstick, which suited her very well, especially when she wore red. She always said what she thought, without mincing words. She gave a lot of help to her large family and relatives and to us, her friends. I will not forget how during our military putsch—the attempt at a military coup in 1991—Betty called several times from Washington and asked worriedly how she—they—could help. Or later, when in Uzbekistan's Ferghana Valley an oil well caught fire, she and Dale did everything they could so that the U.S. government sent the all needed help to prevent an ecological catastrophe. Then, after the collapse of the Soviet Union, she actively helped by sending Russian citizens various kinds of humanitarian aid, including medical equipment and supplies that we needed at the time, strange as that might seem. Betty was a member of the delegation of American women when we were preparing the agenda for the Gorbachev–Bush summit of 1991, "From Disarmament to Kindergartens," and her participation was extremely important for making the main decisions since she knew many members of our delegation and was able to discuss things with us informally. In short, she had become a high-class diplomat yet remained the same modest and polite person she had been before. As I write these reminiscences, my husband, Vadim Repin, who has known Betty for very many years, reminds me how we met her at Domodedovo Airport at night. Betty had been invited by the president of the organization Nevada—Semipalatinsk, the famous poet Oljas Suleimenov, to a ceremony marking the closure of a nuclear testing site in Semipalatinsk [in Kazakhstan, Central Asia]. I was acquainted with him and had suggested that Betty be included among the invited American guests. Betty flew with a stopover in Moscow. But the flight out to Semipalatinsk was delayed several times, and she had phoned us from the airport. I immediately went there and was stunned to see her sitting in a draft and not even in the VIP section. She hadn't even dreamed of requesting this, though she had the right as an invited foreign guest and as the wife of a senator from another country. At that time there were food shortages in Moscow, and Vadim quickly brought us some food and a bottle of vodka to warm up. In this way we sat there all together until the plane took off, and that delay gave us one more opportunity to spend time with Betty and get to know her better. . . . Each time I visit America—and during the past eighteen years this has been often since the family of my daughter, Lala Cornelius, lives in Nashville—I phone Betty. We always speak frankly and try to share good news. For many years she was a member of the Presidium of the Methodist Church, whose headquarters is located in Nashville, directly across from where my daughter Lala lives. And this gave us the opportunity to meet even more often. Betty actively participates in the campaign to vaccinate children, together with Rosalynn Carter. She is well acquainted with the U.S. health care system and actively supported health care reforms under President Clinton, and this gave us much to talk about. Betty unified us, the women of America and the Soviet Union. And now that the republics that composed the Soviet Union have become independent countries, the links she has forged only get stronger. In any case we try to broaden them. Not long ago, in January of this year, I met Valentina Tereshkova at a friendly dinner organized for the members of the International Women's Forum by our well-known artist Zurab Tsereteli. I passed a greeting to her from Betty Bumpers. Valentina responded in a lively way and inquired about how Betty was doing. She also has the fondest memories about their meetings since, you see, there were later trips to visit us by delegations from Peace Links and our delegations were also in the United States.

When the Berlin Wall fell and the "cold war" ended, a war that so held back the development of our general civilization, it was generally considered that the victory was a result of the exertion of political will of the leaders of the countries. I, on the other hand, share the opinion of those people who believe that it was the citizens of our countries who created the climate that made it impossible for this stalemate to continue. The women's movement is first among these, along with others—although women recipients among Nobel laureates are few. Now, when again governments have begun to build bomb shelters, it is time for us to strengthen our ranks. I have a granddaughter growing up, Lara Cornelius, in the United States and other wonderful girls: Katyusha Doronina and Khloya Langford'd in London, Veronika Generozova in Trieste, Lerochka Gus'kova in Moscow, and many others. I tell them how wonderful it is to take part in the work of all humanity (the words of Faulkner), and I believe that they will strengthen the general chain of peace. And bomb shelters from disuse will be rebuilt into clubs of various sorts. I could write more about Betty, about how she knows and loves painting, especially watercolor, about how she is interested in the history of religion and loves good books. About how she considers the tastiest treat in Moscow to be fresh cucumbers, straight from the garden. But we, her friends, are many, and each of us has reminiscences. I think it would not be out of place to end with my favorite lines of verse, which Boris Pasternak wrote on a book given to my friend from Georgia, Chuka Gudiashvili:

> Jolts and revolutions
> do not clear the path to a new life.
> But rather revelations and kind acts
> from someone's inspired soul. . . .

These words I relate to everyone living in my soul—and to Betty.

NOTE

1. Rosalynn Carter, *First Lady from Plains* (Boston: Houghton Mifflin, 1984), 171.

NINE

Detaching, Returning to Arkansas, and the Future

> I like the small town friendliness of Arkansas and the sense of being in a safe and trusted place again. Robert Frost has said home is the place that, when you go there, they have to take you in. I cannot imagine it being any other way in Arkansas.[1]

CONVERSATIONS WITH BETTY[2]

"One of the things I love most about Arkansas is its size. It is small enough for its problems to be manageable and for people to be able to see the results of their efforts. It is easier in Arkansas than in larger states to pinpoint what needs to be done and then to get through to the person who can do something about it. It is a good place to figure out how things happen in a democracy and to see how one person, by taking action or speaking out, can make a difference.

"I do not find the negativism and apathy among people in Arkansas that I often run into elsewhere. The minds of the people here are as open as the spaces they live in. Arkansans tend to be hopeful and optimistic. Because they are used to solving their own problems, they consequently see national problems as capable of being worked out in the same way. They do not view national or international affairs from a 'gloom and doom,' fatalistic perspective such as is found in some quarters. They respond pragmatically and with the attitude that a solution will be found.

"It is that spirit of believing that things can be done, and it is that spirit which accounts, I believe, for the unusual number of leaders Arkansas has produced in the business world, in public life and in arts and literature. The number of Arkansans who have gained national prominence for what they are doing is far greater than would be expected from our percentage of the national population. Such leadership is no accident. Somewhere along the way whatever it is that keeps the spirit up and going seems to be readily available here.

"I'm not suggesting that Arkansans haven't experienced their share of hardships. Some Arkansas families, including my own, made it through the depression years only with great difficulty, and poverty has continued to be a fact of life for too many of us. Despite the hardships, however, or possibly because of them, we have retained our sense of community especially in rural areas and have hung on to the belief that we are our neighbor's keeper. The value system instilled in us by many years of Sunday School remains intact.

"Whenever my plane touches down in Little Rock or Fort Smith, I have the sense of well-being which comes with knowing I am once again home. I know that I will not make it to the luggage area without seeing half a dozen familiar faces and I find that immensely comforting and reassuring."[3]

Dale and I had talked about living in Arkansas in our retirement. The main reason we stayed in Bethesda for several years after Dale retired is that two of our kids and five of our seven grandchildren lived there. Dale, Brooke, and Bill were all in law firms right downtown, so the three met for lunch at least once a month. We had a place in Little Rock, our Patio House, and we could go there every weekend if we wanted to. Lots of our friends were in Arkansas, and Brent and his family lived there. Dale went back often to Arkansas to attend things like dedications, but he doesn't like to fly that much.

It was hard to live in Little Rock full-time right after Dale retired because we couldn't go out to eat—or pretty much anywhere else—without being recognized. Dale loved going to stores, especially grocery stores, but he couldn't even buy groceries in Arkansas without people remembering him. I'd go once a month for things like flour, soda, and baking powder. If we went out to eat, we had ten people coming over to chitchat. In Bethesda, we could live pretty independently. I wouldn't dare go out in Little Rock without putting makeup on—looking like a slob wouldn't be okay.

Brooke's family lived right next door in Bethesda. Brooke has an Australian husband and two adorable redheaded children. When Emily was four years old, Callan was in school, and sometimes I couldn't keep up with that little one. Her husband, Gordon, grew up in Australia until he was fifteen. He went to the University of Colorado and lost a lot of his Australian accent, but the kids have picked up some of it. When Brooke's oldest boy started second grade, he still said, "Well, I cahn't." Here was this rough-and-tumble, rowdy kid that had really more of a Southern accent, I guess, but I heard a few things slip out like, "Well, I cahn't do it." One day he said, "I'm very pleased with my teacher, and so is my mum." He called Brooke "Mum."

When we were in Bethesda, every morning Dale always grabbed the crossword puzzle, and I'd say, "I don't know why you don't let me have it or at least share it. Let me do it every other day." But he didn't; he'd start it in the morning and then take it with him. I had to read that section of the paper first because he'd take the front page first. He'd take the crossword and work on it while he rode the Metro or finish it coming home at night.

As we get older, neither one of us deals with stress as well as when we were younger. Everyday chores seem bigger and more stacked up than they used to. When I get overstressed, I can't sleep. Like one night back in Bethesda, I just fell into bed because I was exhausted, and I didn't even wash my face. But at three o'clock, there I was, wide eyed and bushy tailed. So I went downstairs, drank a glass of milk, and played Freecell, a computer card game, for about an hour. I figured that it helped keep my brain cells active. Dale played Freecell on a handheld video game system. You know who else did that? Hillary Clinton. She and Dale always talked about what speed they operated on and so forth. When Dale got overstressed, that's how he would relax. He would play it because you can't think of anything except trying to move those little things down. I know that's the reason they both turned to video games because when you get overstressed, your mind doesn't even work well.

After Brooke and her family moved to Little Rock, we considered moving more. Brooke lives in a nice neighborhood, and we thought about buying a house in that neighborhood, but it didn't work out. Near her house is a park with a stream running through the middle of it, and her kids like to play there. Dale had a fit about Brooke's allowing her two children to go to the park alone and told her, "I never would have let you children play in such a place alone." Brooke said, "Mom would have." Dale is sometimes ridden with angst. If I got as pessimistic as he did or worried like that about kids playing in the park, we'd have been in trouble. I looked for a place in Little Rock because I kept telling Dale that we needed to come back home while we were still able to. We didn't want to come back in a box. He resisted the move because he liked to go to lunch at the Senate building and see his colleagues.

"In 2008, I spent most of the summer beginning the move to a new house in Little Rock. The hot water tank in the Patio House flooded the place about the same time I found the house I wanted and needed. It was just right for us to retire to, so I bought it. I slowly moved into the new house and fixed up the Patio House for sale. We worked toward Dale retiring at the end of that year.

"In 2009, I was out of touch with old friends most of the year while I was busy getting rid of Bethesda stuff and moving everything to Arkansas. The spurts of moving things were interrupted a few times by health problems for me or for Dale, by doing repairs on the Bethesda house, and by getting out of things I've been involved in for thirty-five years. I felt like a yo-yo. We scheduled the final move during Thanksgiving week. We kept the Bethesda house with skeleton furnishings until the spring housing market. That seemed to be the only way Dale could make the break, and that was okay with me, too, since I couldn't seem to get everything done. Our son Bill lived nearby and took care of things."[4]

People asked me constantly how the senator was adjusting to retirement, and I told them, "I think he is doing just fine. I'm the one who's having a problem getting used to a twenty-four/seven husband—that I did not anticipate."

"I watched all of Barack Obama's inaugural events from my new 'digs' when we were moving to Arkansas. I thought, 'Are we not blessed to have lived, especially me, to see this new president, Barack Obama? I am so happy and just hope he can fulfill a portion of the promise he holds.'"[5]

Later on, I had a call from the White House about President Obama's Afghanistan surge speech. Tina Chen, who works in a White House office—I think it's called the Office of Public Response—called me. I said that I didn't see the whole speech but that I understood what he said. She said they wanted to know what I thought because I am a peace activist. I said I was so glad that he didn't just jump into it, the way Bush jumped into the war in the first place. I was glad that President Obama deliberated about it. I said I trusted him, although I'm disappointed in his decision. I told her I thought he should consider a draft or, if not that, a war tax on the rich. I said, "We've been there eight years, and it's everybody's war now. Everybody should have a stake in it. With the military like it is, this is a poor man's war." She felt that a draft would be too controversial, and I said they should start a war tax then. I think she called me because I was on the board of the U.S. Institute of Peace. Now I'm only on its advisory committee because I've been off the board of directors for several years.

I wish I were in Obama's cabinet right now. I would love to help him when he talks about cutting out waste and programs that don't work. He should look at the ones that do work, like the Agricultural Extension. Extension people do many things that help to establish communities. Back then, it was done with canning kitchens and teaching women how to be good homemakers and how to thrive in a community. A community's needs and direction change all the time. So we need a master organization that's already out there, all over the United States. Extension ladies have stayed ahead of things because, well, they are women. And they recognize that they are trying to help address issues like teen mothers and teen pregnancy by working with families. They've fulfilled that mission so well that they have worked themselves out of a job, and they need a new mandate. They could be the people who oversee the quality of institutions like hospitals and nursing homes. What we need are local people, not only for nursing homes but also for hospitals and other institutions that need to be held accountable.

I went to a 2010 meeting with the Every Child By Two (ECBT) Board, which meets twice a year. ECBT has been the major organization speaking out against the autism scare. Now that it has the data showing that immunization isn't related to autism, I gave them a sermon about getting back to our main mission of making sure that children are immunized on time. We need to just apply Dr. Paul Offit's admonition to "look at the data." Dr. Offit is a vaccine researcher, serves on our ECBT board, and has publicized research to show that immunization has no link to autism. Rosalynn Carter and I want to move to a more globalized effort to immunize children. We are involved with the Gates Foundation, and I work with that sometimes when I am in Bethesda. Amy Pisani, our ECBT executive director, has worked very hard; she has a fabulous office, and I go down there sometimes. I'm also on the board of Vital Voices, which works with women and leadership.

Being an adult retiree volunteer is an awesome responsibility. I volunteer with Life Quest of Arkansas, a program for seniors at a Presbyterian church. Now I do different volunteer things, when I have a chance, things that don't require me to be on a schedule. Our church feeds homeless people, and I'll make a big casserole or take food there whenever I want. The community gathers food for the church's feeding stations. They even accept leftovers after Thanksgiving since it's all about feeding the homeless. I also rock babies at Children's Hospital. Once you are screened, you can come in anytime and play with the babies that are in long-term care.

In Little Rock, we have seen a lot of changes to the downtown area lately, and it has grown a lot. A twenty-story condo building is under construction, and there are real changes for the better along the river near the Clinton Library. There's a story about the time that Lady Bird Johnson came to visit Little Rock and stayed near the downtown and the river. She said, with that Texas accent, that she couldn't believe that beautiful river front was such a mess. She thought we could have such a lovely park down there. It wasn't long before plans were made to clean up the riverfront. We have five pedestrian bridges across the Arkansas River around Little Rock, and the one near Riverfront Park is going to be developed into another walking bridge soon. One bridge has a dam, and the kids love to say that they are walking across the big dam bridge.

The Clinton Library and the Heifer International Project complex are located in Riverfront Park, where old warehouses used to be and have really opened up the area. The city put in the trolley that goes all around downtown and out to the Clinton Library. Riverfront Park, the trails along the river, the amphitheater, and the River Market have brought in a lot of tourists. People visit exhibits at the Clinton Library, and that is where Bill Clinton has all of his papers. I'm proud of the Clinton School of Public Service, which is housed in a wonderful old railroad building near the library. Near that, the Heifer Project building is a LEED [Leadership in Environmental and Ecological Design] platinum-rated building that shows how we could really build green in this country.

I like the River Market farmers' market. It's best on the weekend, though it's hard to find parking. But everybody says I have parking magic because I always find a place. In the fall, you can still get cantaloupe, and I test the melons because I don't like to get a mushy one. I buy okra because Dale and I like it stewed. Sometimes I buy a lot of beans or okra, blanch them, and then freeze them. I usually try to get local tomatoes, but sometimes late in the season they're just from the delta. I buy gourds to use for decorating the house and sometimes get an extra big gourd to make into a birdhouse.

When we take a ride from Little Rock to Fayetteville through the foothills of the Ozarks, it is a gorgeous trip. Mount Magazine, a long mountain at the beginning of the Ozarks, is the tallest peak in Arkansas. That's where the Rockefellers had a working farm, and we always said, "It's what God would have done if she'd had the money." The Rockefellers owned practically the whole top of Mount Magazine. There's a state park there now, Mount Magazine Park, with camping, cabins, and a lodge.

After Mount Magazine and the Ozarks are foothills and the Arkansas River valley, where Altus has developed into a major wine region. Wiederkehr's winery has a fabulous restaurant, and after I became an adult, one of the few times I ever drank a little too much was in 1967 when we came to its grand opening. I had never had much experience with wine; none of us had until wine drinking became a phenomenon in Arkansas and all over the country. My two sisters and a number of us had a reservation at the restaurant, and they served muscadine wine from a grape that grows around here. We had a couple of wild vines of it on our farm, and I remember just loving those muscadine grapes. Oh, and I thought that wine was so tasty. That was the second time in my life that I drank so much I realized I couldn't easily stand up and walk. The first time was at a wedding reception where we were drinking champagne. Dale almost had to help me to the car to get home. Muscadine wine has a distinct flavor, and it is still one of Wiederkehr's most popular wines, even after all these years. Widerkehr's is one of two family wineries in Altus; the other is Post. Both were established in the 1880s, and it is amazing that they are still in the families after so many years.

Ozark is where Brooke and Bill both were born. Charleston is only seventeen miles away, but Ozark is a bigger city and had the hospital. A lot of tornadoes have struck the area around Fort Smith and Charleston, and Brooke was always afraid of them. We called that area, which is near Oklahoma, Tornado Alley. A few years ago, a tornado wiped out a lot of the historic district in Little Rock. Fort Smith was pretty well wiped out by tornadoes twice; in 1927, a little after I was born, the historic district along Garrison Avenue was destroyed. A lot of settlers went out West from there, and the Trail of Tears also went through town and on into Oklahoma. The removal of the Indians from eastern lands was a sad part of the region's history.

Except for my family losing my brother from heart problems at forty-two, all the rest of us are pretty good survivors. My brother would be over ninety now, but he died young. Three of his children are still living, and three died early, as he did, because of our family health problems related to heart disease and high cholesterol. Maggie, the oldest sister, lived into her mid-eighties, although she was in poor health and in the nursing home at the end. I was eighty-seven in January 2012, and my younger sister is in her eighties now. Dale and I both are so lucky that we are still going, but we both had long-lived parents. My mother and dad were both eighty-eight and with clear minds when they died, and so I'm hoping that I make it to eighty-eight—well, shoot, a little longer than that because they say that an eighty-year-old now is the sixty-year-old of yesteryear. I mean, it's like being sixty when you're in your eighties.

I'm at the stage now where I try to say, "I'll think of it in a minute." I used to say, "I've lost a vocabulary word temporarily." Then it would come back after a few minutes or an hour but be inappropriate to interject. Now I've discovered that sometimes it doesn't come back at all. That's what middle-aged people have got to look forward to.

The older I get, the more I believe in nature versus nurture with kids. I have three wonderful, high-achieving, very successful children. They are well-adjusted people, still married to their first spouses, and they grew up fine during the 1960s, so we feel very fortunate. They've never given us any serious problems. They're all good, conscientious people, environmentalists, lawyers, very generous in their giving. They feel a responsibility to others. I'd love to take credit for it, but I just think most of it is in the good gene mix. I think that as parents, we enhance what they're going to be. As I live and observe children, it seems some kids raise themselves or turn out well in spite of their parents. It's hard to grow up nearly as well, though, without nurturing and attention.

There are some things that too many parents don't spend enough time paying attention to or teaching their children that require a stay-at-home mother, I think, or at least a very observant and committed parent. I am not putting down women who work because I know a lot of women have to work. And I am not saying that every mother should be a stay-at-home mother, but I know that if they work, sometimes they don't have time to be that closely observant and patient. They can't be present all of the time to pay that level of attention to their kids.

But I still think that is one reason I have three wonderful, balanced children. I am not bragging; they probably tried drugs—they tried everything—but they had the good sense not to go too far, not to get strung out. We would probably have tried that too, Dale and I both, but as my dad said, "At least they all had a measuring stick and knew when to quit." Of course, thank God, none of them had the genes for addiction, which I do think has a genetic factor. They also had some kind of gumption, or reasoning, to figure out, "Hey this is not for me. This is stupid."

I always said to them, "For God's sake, don't drink until you're not in control because when you are not in control, you don't know what is going to happen to you." And sometimes I just tried to scare the hell out of them—to tell you the truth—about drugs and about drinking. I didn't want them to be goodie-two-shoes or a puss that wouldn't try anything because I tried drinking, and I smoked for thirty years.

Sometimes it's hard to remember all those things that kids need to be told. I have found that even to this day I use information I learned from my mother and dad. My mother used to give good advice when we did something wrong, made a mistake, or failed at something. If we spilled something, she would say, "Oh don't fret about it, wipe it up and go on." That means don't be overcome by failure, by a mistake, or by something bad—use it to learn. Learn something from it and go on. I used that with my own children when they'd do something wrong. So many children don't have anybody who ever says those things to them, but that is what a lot of parenting is all about. That's why I'm a really strong advocate of stay-at-home mothers.

If I could write a scenario that I think would be perfect, it would be for a parent to stay at home with a baby until the child is five and ready for kindergarten, ready to reach out to the world. When children come home and say, "Mother, the teacher doesn't do it that way," they are ready for outside experience. Ideally, a mother needs to be at home teaching and listening to kids play. That is another role of parenting, and I think it's helped me raise three really good kids plus several in the neighborhood who hung around with us.

Working parents can make time, like my daughter and her husband, who both work. Brooke and Gordon read to their children every night. They don't just come home and put the children to bed. They spend the time when they are home reading stories, lying by the children at night, talking until they go to sleep. They are busy, yet they put in good time. That's the strength of this country, I think—good parenting. We have lots of very good parents and some very bad ones.

I always considered it a great privilege to be able to stay at home, and that's not possible for everyone to do. I needed to be working, and I did make sacrifices by staying home. We didn't have any money because of the problems with the hardware store. While it was Dale's own fault, those are faults that paid off. He always has learned everything the hard way, but you know, it's a good way to learn things. Once you've learned those things, they stay with you. If you have any imagination or any foresight, you understand how to use that information. I tell my kids never to shrink from any experience you can have because somewhere down the road in your life, you will use that experience. It may be fifty years from the time you learned it, but it will be information that you will use.

When the kids were growing up and needed discipline, Dale was the good guy—he didn't make a lot of rules. I was the strict parent, the disciplinarian, I guess. I never said, "Wait till you father gets home." I just took care of it, plus I was home more. Of course, Dale expected the children to follow some rules—he was raised with things being black and white, and my family had more gray areas. Brooke has said that she worried because her husband is very easygoing and didn't discipline their kids. She often has to be the bad guy, and she thinks her kids will have bad memories of that. I asked Brooke if she had bad memories of me, and she said no. So I told her not to worry because children need some rules.

Anyway, my children did well, and all finished college in four years. Brent was a skimmer as a student. He would come close to failing, but boy, once he realized he was about to fail, he got in and dug like a crab—and fast—to get himself out of that hole. I think one of the best compliments I ever had was from my son, who was forty-four when he took his newborn twins home. He has a delightful, wonderful wife, my daughter-in-law. I love her, and we get along beautifully. Neither of my daughters-in-law thinks that she has to have mother-in-law trouble like so many young women do. I said to my son one day, when the twins were three, "I need to sit down and have a talk with you and LeAnn about discipline." And he turned and looked at me and said, "Mom, you know I figure that I'm going to parent pretty much the way I was parented. And if LeAnn needs your advice, I think she will ask for it." And I said, "Chalk one up for you, honey—advice well given and well taken."

Brent later made a remark that also helped me. He was talking about people who don't take care of their health, and he doesn't have much patience if they don't take care of themselves. He said, "Well, all of it comes down to parenting—the kind of parenting you had." So I think those are great compliments.

What were my happiest times? I guess that was when we were raising our kids, struggling and raising our kids. But the times now are happy times in my life; I'm just a happy girl. My son Bill was madly in love with a girl one time. He was in law school in Washington, and when he had been here in Little Rock for something, he often would stop to see her on his drive back. Or he would drive down to see her if he had a long weekend from school. One time he came home kind of tired and exhausted, and he asked, "Mom, how do you make a woman happy?"

I said, "Son, let me give you some good advice. You do not make a woman happy. So I want to tell you"—because he was almost thirty years old or in his late twenties—I said, "Marry a happy girl because you don't make someone happy. They are either happy or they are unhappy people. You enhance the happiness, but you don't make them happy."

I tell my husband all the time, even now, "Dale, you choose to be either happy or unhappy. It is your choice, so decide to be happy for God's sakes." I believe in that very strongly, and I just refuse to get bogged down in unhappiness.

I'm also not a complainer or whiner. Brooke has inherited a lot of that; she has hardly ever complained. Her back is fused, and she can't bend over or do a lot of things. But maybe once she did complain. It was when, not long after we had moved to Washington, she had to wear a steel and leather brace. Later, she had one made of plastic and foam that was a little more comfortable. But I had to make her clothes because the brace fit down around her hips; it held her shoulders back and supported her spine to keep it from developing stenosis or scoliosis as much as possible. One time, when she was about thirteen, she complained, "Why did I have to have this?"

And I said, "Brooke, I don't know why you had to have this. And you can hang on a cross for the rest of your life if you choose to, but what you need to concentrate on is the fact that you have loving parents who have done their very best to take care of you. And you have a good mind and will be afforded every opportunity that we possibly can put together for you, so you've got to cope with it." We were driving and had stopped at the light on River Road when a car came by in the turnoff lane. She had her arm out the window, and the car went speeding by and practically sideswiped us.

She jerked her arm in and said, "Jesus Christ! I could have lost my arm!" And she added, "That's all I need, Mom, a gimpy walk and one arm." And do you know, I have never heard her complain about that since. Not one time.

When she was in middle school, she came home one time from an eighth-grade school dance. She has always had a strong ego, and she said, "Why does nobody ever ask me to dance?" You talk about a heart-breaker. I said, "I don't know, honey, but you are looking at the queen of wallflowers. I was never really popular. I always had one boy, maybe—and I always had dates for this, that, and the other—but I was never real flypaper for boys. Boys never paid much attention to me, but look who I ended up with."

Now that we are all in Little Rock, we see Brooke and her family a lot. Both of the children are in school; I pick them up sometimes. They eat at our house a lot because they work. Brooke's husband, Gordon, runs a clinic for indigent women at the medical center. His instructors recommended him for this, as he is appreciative of all women. He also has set up a women's prison program, and he sees some bad conditions and ailments there. He goes twice a week to do preventive medicine, so the women have more than just emergency care. Brooke goes back to D.C. sometimes with her law practice.

We all get together for the holidays. At this time, we don't make a big thing out of birthdays; we usually just call each other. At Christmas, we sometimes play a game called "Dirty Santa." Everybody buys a pretty nice present for maybe twenty or thirty dollars. Sometimes they are funny, but a lot of the time they are just nice gifts. We bring them wrapped, and we put everyone's name into a hat. The first person drawn gets first choice of all the wrapped presents. Then the next person gets to choose, and after they open the gift, they can keep it or trade it for the first one opened. So it keeps going on like that until the person whose name is drawn last gets the choice of the gift they opened or any of the other presents.

I'll tell you, the empty nest is not all good, but it's not all bad, either. I loved watching my children, and I still do love watching my grandchildren, observing them as they learn new things. I like just watching kids on the street, seeing the experiences they have and the light turning on and all. It's fun. That's why people are teachers and why we have so many good teachers; it's because they enjoy the same thing.

My kids teach their children good values. They take them once in a while to church, and they go to church with me some. Brooke takes them more often because she belongs to a church. I chide my children about not going often enough and tell them, "You are remiss in not taking your children to Sunday school and church." But I haven't gotten very far with it. I don't nag them a lot, but I remind them pretty often, "Your children need it. They need to be exposed to the lessons of the church. Even if you teach them those lessons, they are not being reinforced by the church or by other people. People in the church that you belong to will care about your children and want to keep up with them." I kept up with the children in my church, and I still do. I say, "They care about your children, and it is a church home. What do you think that means?"

I remind them, "When you were little, sometimes you said. 'I am smarter than that so and so, my Sunday school teacher.' And I told you back then, 'Yeah, but his heart is in it. He is trying to do something for you. He is part of your church family.'"

The church taught me a lot of wonderful lessons. That's what I tell my children all the time. The teachings of the Ten Commandments and the Sermon on the Mount are valuable reinforcements for what you teach your children. [When the interviewer asked,] I'll say I was never really spiritual. I supported the church as an institution because I knew what good work it did in the community, and I knew what it meant for our well-being and social life as members of the community. The church supported the things we supported: the vacation church schools we had every year, the food baskets we sent for, and the help that we did with the missions, although I never really believed in missions. Even then, I thought, "What business do we have, going into foreign countries trying to change them from the beliefs they have, to our beliefs? Who knows who is right?"

I stayed active in the church because I support the institution, and I believe in it. Yet I look around and see what havoc religion has wreaked in the world. Religions have created some of the worst atrocities, from the Crusades down to right now. The fundamentalists in any religion would chop your head off if they got the chance. The more history I have learned, the more agnostic I have become. I mean, I don't believe in the virgin birth, as some of those birth miracles come from Greek mythology. The more educated you are, the more agnostic you become, in a way, unless you can buy into all that. Faith is just not that big a deal with me; I can't take it all by faith.

However, I am a great believer in prayer because I think that it is just you helping yourself by pausing and thinking about or trying to deal with things you pray about. At night, I try to count my blessings and similar things; a lot of the old traditions are great helps in life. But I don't even like to repeat the Apostles' Creed. At times I just think, "What are you really saying?" As far as the communion, I participate in communion as just a kind of ritual, a role. It's just something I do when I go to church, but it is still important. As I said, I support the institution even if I don't agree with everything.

Over time, I've worked to humble myself because I have been grateful and humbled by the opportunities I have had. I've remembered Methodist Church teachings as well as my mother often reminding us that the only unforgivable sin is the sin of omission. I have used that idea to motivate Senate wives and many other community leaders. If you ignore an opportunity, that is the sin of omission: it's not taking advantage of your ability to do something that would rectify a wrong or help accomplish something. My mother and I equated avoiding those opportunities and chances to sinning—the sin of omission.

A lot of these are lessons I learned in the Methodist Church. The Ten Commandments are things that you can apply to life. I learned about the teachings of Susanna Wesley, for one thing; I read and reread the book about her. Her husband was a preacher and was gone a lot. She was left with twelve children, and she had to educate them and make socially good beings out of them. Her rules and regulations were passed down through the Methodist Church, and my grandmother passed on all kinds of them, like cleanliness is next to godliness. Those things are invaluable to ingrain in a child's head if you can. As a child, you think at the time, "Oh, ho hum." But somehow they are in there and are most valuable.

Other than the well-being of my children and being a support to them, the most important thing now is to grow old with grace. So here is what I strive for now: Try to be pleasant. Try to be positive. Try to be less critical. Try to be less bossy. Try to be more charitable. Trying to be in grace in those ways relates to a description of growing old in grace that I heard once in a sermon. I think of that sermon sometimes and about what grace means; it reminds me of what is important.

People who do yoga talk about being happy and about your mind-set. My yoga instructor the other day was trying to help me get this crick out of my neck—I think it was stress or something. Anyway, he asked, "What is your goal in life?"

To which I said, "At this stage in my life, it is to grow old in grace."

He said, "That's because you already accomplished your goals. I Googled you, and I know."

I said, "You're silly." He is so young, about twenty-five. He makes us take deep breaths and suck in our guts one hundred times. He overworks me, and I sometimes take it out on him by telling him he's silly. But I also told him that I want to grow old in grace.

I would like to be remembered for being a good mother and a good wife and for trying to live up to my beliefs about the sin of omission. That means I hope I have taken advantage of every opportunity that has come along to try to do something worthwhile. Just being a good person, I guess, or as good as I can be, not being thought of as a petty, small-minded person or someone too self-absorbed.

My proudest legacy is my family of three fine children and, hopefully, seven fine grandchildren. I'd like to be remembered as having been as honest and as forthright and as humble as I try to be and not too jaded by all of the opportunities I've had. I want to be remembered as being grateful. More than anything else is to be remembered as being grateful for my heritage and grateful for my luck and my life. When I look back and think, I really have been afforded some fabulous opportunities in my life.

I have been very lucky in that I have had some very serious illnesses and have survived them. I hope to be remembered for my tenacity and spirit to keep going, a lot of which comes from my mother, who often didn't feel well when we were young children. Recently, Dale would be wimping around about not getting out in the cold weather when he had a cold, and he would worry and fuss at me when I had any little thing wrong with me. He'd say, "You ought not to be out there doing this or doing that."

One time I said about my mother, who survived five primary malignancies and was tenacious about fighting for her life, "Dale, do you ever remember my mother going to bed?"

He said, "Come to think about it, I don't think I ever do." And he said that when he had known her his entire adult life.

I said, "You never did see her in bed." And I have told my kids, "If you ever see me take to the bed, you'll know the end is near." I think that is one reason I survived these illnesses that I've had over the years, even the serious ones.

Also, I have always had wonderful friends, so there are so many people who have added to my work. The Sassers, Jim, who was the senator from Tennessee while Dale was in the Senate, and his wife, Mary, are our best friends, and they've toured Russia with us. Joan Baker, who was active in Peace Links, is a good friend and now my neighbor in Little Rock. She traveled with me to Russia, taking vacation time from her work. When she and her husband retired, they traveled and worked with Habitat for Humanity and taught English as a second language in Yugoslavia and Vietnam. Later, when she divorced, she traveled with me to Israel and other places.

Another friend in Little Rock, Sara Murphy, who died years ago, helped write down my thoughts for organizing Every Child by '74, and later she helped with getting Peace Links under way. Nell Balkman taught me about community organizing. Laurie Daschle writes speeches for me. Joycelyn Elders helped to coordinate a lot of the Every Child by '74 campaign as it came together, and we spent a lot of time flying around Arkansas together. Amy Pisani is another. I haven't done any of these things alone—I've had very, very good help.

Looking back now, I see that my early life was a different era. I've watched the TV show by Ken Burns, *The War*. He covers the history of World War II, including the failures. My generation remembers all of that, and Burns's work is a good history lesson. I love the music, too. But sometimes I have to turn it off—I couldn't watch the battles in West Africa and Italy. Dale joined the service in 1941, and later he was headed to Hawaii with a group of marines who were going to be part of the invasion of Japan. When the U.S. dropped the atomic bombs and the war ended, I could only think about how glad I was that he was coming home.

I have no way of judging how well we have covered my life in these interviews; I have participated in so many things. I see a lot of examples of the serendipity of my life. Recently, a young woman came up to me after lunch at a restaurant and said, "Are you my aunt Betty?" It was my niece by marriage, whom I'd never met. She was trying to assemble and computerize national health records. I've worked on that effort for twelve years, trying to get immunizations transferred onto electronic records; Arkansas could be a model for this. And the same day, while we were touring the governor's mansion, I got to talk to the governor [Mike Bebee] and Ginger about electronic health records. It's amazing.

When I talk about the past, sometimes it just seems like a lot of rattle to me. It was kind of olden times, if you think about it. When you're my age, you know you've lived through an era. Then I look back and think that it has been sort of an enchanted life.

CONNECTIONS

CONVERSATIONS WITH JOAN BAKER[6]

I was on the Peace Links National Board. Working with Peace Links and knowing Betty, I can tell you that unlike a lot of political people, Betty has no ego problems. She never cares who gets credit for anything, as long as the goal is accomplished and the work gets done.

Betty and I traveled extensively together. When we traveled to Cuba, we subjected to a long tirade regarding America's faults by a prominent women government official there. When we were traveling in Japan, Betty said, "I used my position shamelessly to promote issues I cared about." The women didn't know what she meant, and it didn't translate at first, so she thought a minute and said, "That's called pillow talk in America." And then they got it!

I was still working with the Peace Links Board when the national office closed. We could see the handwriting on the wall that some of the new Republicans who had been elected to Congress were not going to be interested in our agenda or goals. Fund-raising would prove difficult.

We only had a few wives of Republican members of Congress involved at the last gala. It was our big fund-raiser, and the way it was going, that fund-raising was not going to work. People came to the event to see the members of Congress. Lobbyists could afford the thousand-dollar cost, and they bought the tickets. If there wasn't good congressional turnout, then the lobbyists wouldn't come. In the end, when we closed shop, we gave the Peace Links funds to several other like-minded organizations.

Did anyone tell you about Betty and the Peace Links FBI files? I don't know exactly how Dale and Betty decided to ask, but they could get the files under the Freedom of Information Act. The Peace Links file was about two inches thick, and most of the information was redacted, of course. Now you have to wonder, what would the Federal Bureau of Investigation have had to say about Betty or Peace Links?

The FBI gathering those files about Peace Links was the same sort of thing that happened with Senator Denton. Early in Peace Links's organizing, Senator Jeremiah Denton of Alabama got up on the Senate floor and spoke about Betty and Peace Links. He implied that working with Peace Links or other peace organizations was an unpatriotic thing to do. Several senators defended Betty, and it got Peace Links good free publicity.

"VOICES WE HEARD"

JOAN BAKER
AUGUST 27, 1989

First, I'll give you a little background on my trip. I work for Senator Bumpers of Arkansas, and his wife, Betty, who founded an organization about eight years ago called Peace Links (which now has a membership of over 35,000 members). Pax World Foundation, like Peace Links, is an organization founded to promote international understanding. They invited Betty to make up a group of twenty people to go to Israel and Jordan for two weeks to observe and learn about the Palestinian refugee problem.

Betty gathered an interesting group of people—three Jewish women, one who had been a lifelong Zionist and who remembered as a child having Chaim Weizmann, who is considered to be the father of modern-day Israel, come to her home. Miriam had also been involved in getting Jews out of Germany in 1938 after Kristalnacht. Another Jewish woman on the trip (formerly married to a Hollywood producer) is chairman of the Hollywood Women's Political Committee (one of those wild-eyed liberal organizations). William Sloan Coffin's brother and his wife joined us. She's state chairman of the Democratic Party in Vermont, and he's an international businessman. I believe Dr. Coffin is now head of SANE/FREEZE, a national peace organization. We had a couple from Iowa active in the World Peace Through Law organization. He is a state representative from Iowa. We had an editor of one of the Boston papers and a publicist for the San Francisco Ballet who was Lebanese and whose fluency in the Arab language helped us through some tight situations.

All of us tried to read as much as we could on the subject, we were sent the State Department's basic briefing papers, we were reminded *several* times to go with an open mind—this was to be an evenhanded approach. I read a quote from a journalist who had covered the Middle East for ten years. He said, "First, when it comes to discussing the Middle East, people go temporarily insane, so if you're planning to talk to an audience of more than two, you'd better have mastered the subject." Well, I'll confess, I have not mastered the subject, but I think we did have a fairly good exposure to the situation. This was definitely not a tourist group. We had meetings day and night and did almost no sightseeing. Fortunately, I had been there before a few years ago.

"Israel," "Palestine," "The Holy Land," "The Promised Land," "Judea and Samaria," "The Land of Canaan," "The Fertile Crescent"—whatever you call that tiny speck of land in the Middle East situated between the Jordan River and the Mediterranean Sea, it is a *troubled* land. We, as a group, came back saddened, confused, bewildered, and heartsick at the misery, violence, and degradation we witnessed. I would like to say we also came back hopeful—and there *were* glimmers of hope—but very few.

We met with representatives from all walks of life—Jordanian, Israeli, and Palestinian government officials; writers, doctors, and lawyers; a Supreme Court justice; hospital administrators; nurses; American embassy officials; men, women, and students from various peace organizations; and even a former Israeli general who represented 200 other Israeli Army generals. We met officials from the Middle East Council of Churches and the United Nations Welfare and Relief Agency who are doing what they can to alleviate some of the misery and meet some of the critical needs of the thousands of Palestinians in the refugee camps. We also heard the voices of the people on the street, our bus drivers, our guides, waiters, and the shopkeepers, and they had all been deeply affected by the policies of the Israeli government. The voices were full of despair but also hopeful that peaceful solutions *can* be found. When we asked what we could do as Americans to help, most of them said, "Go back and tell the American people what you have seen and heard."

A bright spot for us was a meeting with Hilla, sixteen, a young Jewish girl, and Samer, seventeen, a Palestinian from East Jerusalem whose family had lived in Jerusalem for over 800 years. They were participants in a Legacy International project with the purpose of bringing together Israeli and Palestinian students to discuss their common problems. They told us they would be coming to Bedford, Virginia, in June for a six-week seminar for training in dialogue techniques between adversaries and then return to Israel to encourage other students to become involved in peacemaking. Samer had finished high school and was anxious to go to the university, but because all the universities open to Palestinians are closed, he will have to wait.

Betty and I had the privilege of going down to Bedford, Virginia, a few weeks ago to observe the Legacy International camp. They had brought together 130 students from cultures in conflict from all over the world—Ireland and Northern Ireland, Soviets and Americans, African, Central Americans, Israelis, and Palestinians. It was fascinating to see how they teach those young people to deal with conflict. I thought it was interesting that the camp solves the problem of the dietary restrictions of the different religions and cultures by maintaining a strict vegetarian diet—they even grow all their own vegetables.

I wish I knew some answers—I wish I knew what to do to help alleviate the suffering in Israel. I have to agree with David Shipler, the *New York Times* correspondent, who said, "There will be no peace in the Middle East until pluralism becomes a spiritual truth." I think we could substitute the word "world" for "the Middle East" in that phrase—"there will be no peace in the *world* until pluralism becomes a spiritual truth." All faiths and all people *must* learn to live and let live, and we *must* all continue to "light a candle in the darkness." I believe one way to do that is to continue to make the effort to become informed on the issues. I am convinced that informed, intelligent, compassionate people can and will come up with the bold ideas and initiatives necessary to find peace.

NOTES

1. Betty Bumpers, "Why I Like Arkansas," manuscript and correspondence with Bob McCord, May 6, 1986, Peace Links Records (MC 907) series 1, subseries 1, box 2, folder 2-9, Special Collections, Unviersity of Arkansas Libraries, Fayetteville, 1–2.
2. Materials within quotation marks are from Bumpers's speeches or writings, cited as endnotes below. Materials outside quotation marks are derived from interviews with Betty Bumpers by Anna and Jennie Eblen, August 29–31, 2005; May 14, 2006; October 2–6, 2007; and February 24–26, 2009.
3. Bumpers, "Why I Like Arkansas."
4. Betty Bumpers, e-mail, 2008–2009.
5. Betty Bumpers, e-mail, 2009.
6. Conversations with Joan Baker occurred in Little Rock, Arkansas, February 24–26, 2009, and are reconstructed from Anna Eblen's field notes, with assistance from Joan Baker. Following these field notes are excerpts from "Voices We Heard," Ms. Baker's contributed essay on her trip to Israel with Betty Bumpers and others.

TEN

Understanding a Life Story

Anna L. Eblen and Colleen Kelley

> Women approach the struggle for peace with a passion and determination which make it impossible for their voices to be ignored. . . . We acknowledge the fact that we tend to think relationally and to see the world as interconnected.[1]

Throughout this book, Betty Bumpers offers personal insights about her intentional communication strategies as she describes using colloquial expressions effectively, tapping into community networks, daring to speak up, using her influential political position, employing appeals to women's ways of knowing, advancing idealism, and relying on tenacity to carry through her work. However, as communication and feminist scholars, we can further assess the layered symbolism of her words and work and help evaluate long-term effects of her social change efforts. For perspective on her social change efforts, we offer a close reading of the materials collected in this volume.

In the communication discipline, we examine the ways that people create meaning from experience. We assume that underlying meanings are important, that patterns in language reveal meaning, and that we can detect and identify patterns. In the following discussion, we explore Bumpers's use of imagery and myth, with special attention to her memories about growing up on a farm. We seek to illuminate how she managed cultural values, especially how she dealt with contradictory ideas about women. Finally, we position her work in an overview of social changes around the issues of immunization and peace. Scholars of oral history,[2] linguistics,[3] rhetoric,[4] and feminist theory[5] inform our reflections and conclusions.

In our final reflections, we return to earlier questions: How does Betty Bumpers perceive the influences of people, places, and events? How do language patterns in her stories reveal the meanings that Bumpers finds in her life? How can we better understand the lives of women by understanding Bumpers's experiences growing up and as Arkansas First Lady and Senate wife? How should we evaluate Bumpers's main contributions to society?

IMAGERY AND MYTHS

A person's life story often has elements of personal myth that may combine with a cultural myth[6] from the times, places, and people encountered. According to Yow, renowned oral historian, personal myths can organize an individual's inner life and integrate personality with events, past and present.[7] Rushing, theorist of rhetoric, defines cultural myth as "a society's collectivity of persistent values, handed down from generation to generation."[8]

"Myths are not necessarily imaginary stories or fables, but can be imbedded in the very language of a culture."[9] Myths portray crucial values that allow people to create and read meanings, just as Bumpers's story represents her thoughts on the meaning of her experience. Bumpers does not just list facts but chooses words and a story line that best represent how she has come to understand herself and what has happened. In Bumpers's life, growing up on the farm is a personal myth that evokes the American frontier myth.[10] Bumpers shows a powerful ability to demystify the frontier myth's dangerous aggression and excessive individualism. She highlights instead the frontier myth as courageous building of communities, with recognition of the interconnections that sustain the land, ecosystems, and inhabitants.

The farm stands as a powerful symbol in the American frontier myth. It is a good place for Bumpers to begin her story because the "log cabin" represents the home of extended family, the beginning of a community, and taming of the wilderness. Bumpers presents the farm as the first and dominant story line when describing her life. "I grew up on a farm" has become her starting point in most interviews and many speeches.[11] This prominent, consistent language implies that the farm has become more than a literal place in her life, and its symbolism links with at least three important parts of her life story. First, the farm symbolizes the family itself, with details about the personalities and lives of her family revealed through descriptions of the farm. Second, the farm has come to mean Betty's growing up, as she says, "I grew up on a farm." Third, the farm sets the scene for stories about values: hard work, resourcefulness in difficult times, community, and democracy.

When the farm symbolizes family, Bumpers connects the land to her description of her parents and grandparents. She remembers depletion of the land as a reason her father began to trade cattle, underlining difficulties in making a living there. She relates that the farm's isolation and hard work accounts for her mother's determination to move away. Almost as an afterthought, she adds the fact that her father did not like farming. The farm also figures in her account of her affectionate relationship with her grandparents. She recalls working with her grandfather Flanagan on his farm and stopping in after school at their house adjacent to her parents' farm.

When the farm symbolizes growing up, Bumpers tells stories about sustenance from the land. She vividly describes the food produced there, especially the food that she ate as a child. In the literal sense, food was an issue for many families during the Great Depression, the farm supplied nourishment, and people's connections to farms and farmers fed many. Food, however, also symbolizes love. Those who fed her were also those who loved her, and Bumpers's memories link food and affection. Those who gardened and prepared the food literally helped Betty grow. The power of the food images combined with Bumpers's loving tone evokes extraordinary sensory experiences. Her statement "*That* was food" implies that everyday food cannot compete with the farm's mythic tastes, textures, and aromas.

The farm in Bumpers's life myth also symbolizes interconnections and values, foreshadowing her later activist work. The farm stories showed hard work and resourcefulness. Because it was the location of various cooperative community endeavors, the farm also symbolizes the appropriate relationship of neighbors, emphasizing community. Bumpers reports the shared making of sorghum molasses at her father's press and the threshing machines and workers that moved across the community—from field to field. The products and food of the farm were shared with the community, especially those in need. The farm in Bumpers's myth also provides a setting that shows democratic values and the appropriate relationship of citizens with their government. Bumpers extolled the Extension Service, a federal and regional program that taught farming and homemaking techniques. Aspects of the farm signify community as well as individuality and self-sufficiency. In the frontier myth, over time a community grows around the farm that stands at the edge of the wilderness; Bumpers's experience of the New Deal became a part of her understanding of government's role in developing communities and supporting individual effort.

LANGUAGE PATTERNS, GENDER, AND PARADOX

Bumpers also tells stories of the farm as mythic setting when she discusses gendered roles, such as father and mother, to illustrate cultural values. In childhood, Bumpers absorbs aspects of both roles, but later in life she strategically deploys the mother role most extensively. In her talk, mother has simultaneous and sometimes paradoxical meanings: It is the literal fact of being mothered and mothering in her own life, a metaphor for caring and protection. Mothering is also a contested frontier myth role—images that emphasize homebound caretaker contrast with pioneer women journeying in new directions. Sometimes the frontier myth is so masculinized that mothers are invisible, and Bumpers has a special talent for rebalancing the myth by retelling the story and reminding us that women pioneered alongside men.

Women struggle with the myth and contradictions inherent in symbols such as mother, and feminist theorists explore these cultural ambiguities. Taylor and Perry discuss "paradoxes" as gendered definitions that appear mutually exclusive yet include "sufficient truth that neither can be dismissed."[12] According to Taylor and Perry's analysis of paradox, women can learn to recognize such contradictions, understand their implications, and adopt a "both/and" philosophy for dealing with them. Paradox can inspire creativity and cultural understanding.[13] For Betty Bumpers, this included embracing the many definitions of symbols like "parent (mother/father) and child (daughter/son)" as well as gender-based concepts of "work and play" or "health and illness." She found creative ways of managing contradictions.

For example, Bumpers calls her childhood Arkansas society "chauvinistic," which indicated that, as an elder, she recognized limitations that were problematic for women and girls, who faced restrictive gender role norms. Conservative "frontier" elements of American culture maintained strong hierarchies that placed men above women and parents above children.[14] Simultaneously, progressive elements, such as the New Deal programs, influenced the family and American society. These paradoxes may have been especially important because Bumpers identified with both parents, and despite their patriarchal gender roles, she learned to question hierarchy, gendered division of labor, and the impact of gender on health and well-being.

Bumpers related stories from the farm showing that her parents encouraged a more flexible gender role approach for their children if not for themselves. Her parents modeled roles that seemed traditionally "masculine" for her father and "feminine" for her mother. According to her narrative, Bumpers values both of her parents' teachings, although she seems to identify with her parents in different ways. She identified with her father's speaking patterns, political ideas, and colloquial humor. She admired his strong-willed qualities, even some chauvinistic habits that might have caused difficulties for the women in his life. At the same time, Bumpers provides details that show she also identified with her mother, especially her mother's education, energy, and homemaking skills.

Along with traditional roles, the Flanagan family had a pragmatic model that allowed their young girls to be "treated like men" when farmwork had to be done. This convinced at least one of the daughters that the Flanagans "could do anything . . . if we work hard enough." This model produced paradoxes centered on gender and work, beginning in Bumpers's childhood and continuing throughout her life story. She adapted to paradox by frequently disregarding stereotyped work roles herself while acknowledging their importance to others.

Conservative and progressive models disagree regarding gender-appropriate work.[15] Bumpers refers to "men's work" as she describes the tasks that needed to be done on the farm. She also notes that she preferred this outdoor work and her sisters liked working inside. Additionally, her father's cattle trading business flourished, and Bumpers took on roles shared only by her brother and some hired men when she helped transport cattle and joined the auctions. Bumpers saw the following work paradoxes as worthy of comment in her oral history interviews: her mother's resistance to overwhelming housework and child care, Bumpers's choices to do outside farming and men's work, her sister Ruth's unwillingness to sew, and her brother's ability to do the men's work of farming and women's work of quilting. Bumpers's acknowledgment of gendered work paradoxes particular to their family suggests that these were not taken for granted in 1930s Arkansas culture.

Bumpers describes a health and illness paradox in her discussion of how her well-educated mother, Ola, complained of severe headaches as she handled the role of farmhouse wife. Bumpers implies that her mother's ill health was not only attention seeking but also a response to the strains of childbearing, child rearing, and the never-ending housework and farmwork. While resting or shirking tasks might not have been acceptable ways of dealing with fatigue, poor health had its advantages. When Ola was ill, she sometimes received special treatment. Furthermore, Bumpers' elder sister Maggie had a heart ailment, and, in the opinion of her sister, often used it to avoid her share of the work.

This is not to say that Ola's and Maggie's illnesses were less than real but merely to point out that sickness has symbolic value as well as literal manifestations and consequences. Others have written about the physical manifestations of stress and particularly of the symbolic representations of illnesses that affect women. In the Victorian era, the Cult of the True Woman influenced a generation of women whose paradoxical experiences led to various forms of frailty and illness.[16] Although she often felt bad, Ola used her education and energy to protect her children's health. Bumpers said that her mother knew about nutrition and cleanliness as ways to avoid sickness. Ola kept the children well despite her own health issues. However, the need to deal with the paradoxes of their mother's and sister's poor health led Betty and Ruth to regard illness negatively and try hard never to appear sick.

World War II was remarkable for changes within gender roles when young men departed for the military and young women filled jobs that were left short of workers. Bumpers and her sister took over the dairy bar jobs of two male cousins. Gender paradoxes were involved in decisions to spend her college years at Iowa State and the Chicago Academy of Fine Arts as well as her choice of college major. Although she first wanted to study landscape architecture, Bumpers found that she was the only woman in the classes and the major, so she changed majors. Later, Bumpers specialized in fashion design at the Chicago Academy of Fine Arts. As she became more independent from her family, she perceived a strong possibility of accomplishment in fashion and design, but her father redirected her. Bumpers's decisions appear to have been affected by the paradoxes about gender-appropriate work manifested in the "men-only" major and her father's advice about a career that he saw as inappropriately "tough" for her.

Although she tells these stories in a humorous tone, her father's maneuvering during her teen years illustrates his patriarchal privilege and the double standard about work life. For example, it was the right of her father to move the family for his work despite their (perhaps unvoiced) objections. The double standard of proper female behavior was enforced when her father removed Maggie and Ruth from their sweethearts in the family move to Iowa for his work. Bumpers joked that both sisters had married their beaus anyway. Later, her father's negative comments about her proposed career in fashion design influenced Bumpers's decision not to pursue her interests.

Bumpers also faced gender paradoxes in the postwar era when popular culture urged middle-class women to drop their jobs and return to homemaking. Media messages after the war centered on a return to some aspects of the Cult of the True Woman.[17] While many women exited the public sphere of work for the private sphere of home, they often did so reluctantly. When she and Dale married and returned to Charleston, Betty taught school. She commented on several gender paradoxes, especially when it came to the life of a married teacher, with personal and financial sacrifices whether she taught or stayed home. Opposing cultural values around career and home intensified when Bumpers had children. For instance, if she wanted to work as an elementary school teacher during her pregnancies, she was required to hide the physical changes from students and colleagues. She successfully did so twice but remarked on the paradox of the education system's supposed high regard for families and simultaneous negativity about childbearing.

Career and homemaking also had paradoxical sacrifices and benefits. The benefit of a woman's potential income was seen as coming at the price of her family's well-being. Bumpers says that they really needed her financial contribution from teaching, but she also discloses the costs of this contribution, including less time with her own children and nuisances or expenses of outside child care. Bumpers perceived paradox when the demands of child rearing disallowed time for herself and her interests. She contrasted excitement in career work with frequent boredom in child-rearing work; childrearing was important work yet tedious at times.

The gendered health/illness paradox manifested anew during Bumpers' teens and early adulthood, and these ordeals brought Bumpers to new understandings around health issues. Bumpers's decision to leave college reintroduced health and illness to her story. She goes into some detail about the appendectomy that led to her withdrawal from Iowa State. Later, maturing recognitions about health perhaps provided insights needed to deal with her daughter's life-threatening illness. When Brooke became gravely ill, the family focused on her recovery. Once again, the story showed attention to female illness, but this episode was less about gender and more about heroic family efforts. Bumpers expressed protective mothering and gendered caretaking during years of physical therapy with her daughter. This experience may have helped Bumpers accept a new advocacy challenge when the family moved to the governor's mansion.

REFLECTIONS ON BUMPERS'S SOCIAL CHANGE CONTRIBUTIONS

Bumpers's most renowned work as First Lady of Arkansas involved an early childhood immunization program, the first of her several efforts. She handled this issue creatively, appealing for the protection of children. She promoted the cause of children's health within mothering norms that were acceptable to traditional or progressive Arkansas families who agreed on a moral obligation to protect their children's health.[18] Bumpers navigated the Arkansas political forces carefully but stretched the boundaries of the usual political wife's volunteer work. She went beyond ladylike support and actively mobilized resources throughout the state for the campaign. When Dale was elected to the U.S. Senate, Betty found that her expertise from the Arkansas immunization campaign moved her activism into the national arena. Her work in Arkansas became a model for immunization around the United States.

Continuing her national immunization work with U.S. First Lady Rosalynn Carter, Bumpers soon felt moved to protect children in yet another way. During the early 1980s nuclear proliferation, she encountered contradictory norms as she engaged the war/peace paradox. These included attempts to silence women in the public sphere and the peace movement's need for appropriate, effective persuasion as well as the need to implement nonviolent protest.

The pivotal event in Bumpers's peace movement awakening was as a mother interacting with her daughter, Brooke. The story, told and retold, took on a special meaning within Peace Links. Mothers' responses to children's nuclear war fears resonated so profoundly that women identified their own "Brooke story." Recitations of these stories enlivened Peace Links gatherings and literature, suggesting the literal mothering experience along with significant cultural symbolism. However, there is a significant debate on the use of the mother symbol, especially in advocacy for peace.

Regarding motherhood, peace, and conflict, we find numerous symbolic positions. Feminists criticize use of the mother symbol when it encourages women's restriction to the private sphere (the home), as the most conservative models require. Feminists also resist the implication that mothering (in the sense of reproduction and nurturance) or peacefulness are "natural" roles for women, with implications that all women share similar experiences of mothering or that other roles for women are not natural and that peacefulness is not natural for men. There are also recurring questions about mothers who willingly sacrifice themselves or their children to ideologies. In this case, the contested symbol is protective mothering that sends offspring to defend the dominant group, state, or religion. In a competing position, middle-class peace activists, including Peace Links, define mothering as safeguarding children's safety and sense of security.

In the feminist critique, "mothering" is more than reproduction and must include non-Western definitions. It includes alternative family structures and "fierce" protective mothering to resist corrupt authority.[19] Other theorists expand the metaphor to include forms of caring; for instance, caring is advancing novices who need encouragement in political action.[20] Bumpers's women's leadership work highlights this sort of mentoring. The feminist debate questions the extent to which social movements can use compelling symbols, such as the mother, to their advantage without evoking counterproductive meanings. The more paradoxes that are intertwined with the symbol, the more counterproductive meanings the symbol may evoke. In the nuclear freeze movement, however, paradoxes in Bumpers's mother metaphors aligned with paradoxes about mainstream/radical appeals in the overall campaign.

Appeal to a mainstream audience was one of the nuclear freeze goals. The movement eschewed violence; "fighting" for peace is an ethical contradiction. Bumpers's protective mother metaphor fit well within this movement; it hearkened to mainstream values while standing up against dangers to children inherent in nuclear proliferation. Lofland speaks of "the paradox of polite protest": Although citizens striving for global peace and justice over the 1980s formed a social movement, they mostly refrained from engaging in "abrasive protest or violence of a seriously threatening nature." Instead, they revealed civility and restraint. "While its protest was paradoxically polite, its idealistic and even radical goals tagged it as a social movement that has persisted for generations."[21] Bumpers's Peace Links belonged to an era of antinuclear activism that has been seen by some as less effective because, for ethical reasons, it lacked the radical flank effect.[22] Lofland disagrees and suggests that the 1980s peace movement organizations were more often than not effective precisely because they opted for polite protests rather than threats.[23]

An additional characteristic of the 1980s peace associations, particularly those oriented to citizen diplomacy, was the tendency for the democratic groups that were substantially dependent on a handful of charismatic volunteers to become "mom-and-pop shops"; in this parallel to the mother metaphor, a local couple or individual occupied a central role. Often these individuals became not only the organizers of the group but also the reason for the group's existence. Peace Links represented a particular version of the nuclear freeze–era peace organization formation, the "focusing figure organization" with emphasis on "the moving spirit in her or his circle."[24]

Betty Bumpers became inseparable from the Peace Links organization, both at its founding, initially as a loose coalition of seven state coordinators who assisted women's groups, and in its later development. Many early Peace Links were political wives, often expressing concern for their children. Although Peace Links, such as governors' wives Dorothy Lamm of Colorado and Sharon Percy Rockefeller of West Virginia as well Niki Tsongas, wife of Senator Paul Tsongas, were connected through marriage and ideology to the Democratic Party, the organization was bipartisan. However, despite the political pedigree of Peace Links, Bumpers and the group were attacked as "dupes" of communism both on the floor of the U.S. Senate and elsewhere. In this gender paradox drama, male authority denied women's right to operate in the public sphere and their intellectual ability to argue public policy. For some political wives, this controversy encouraged their determination to extend their advocacy; Bumpers and her associates relished the debate.

Lofland argues that a major characteristic of peace associations organized around citizen action is their "soar-and-slump dynamic," a rapid onset and rise after which comes a decline.[25] The Peace Links organization became virtually indistinguishable from Betty Bumpers's persona and discourse during its early surge. Many factors in the mid- to late 1980s produced public perceptions of a relatively stable world (compared to the perils identified during the nuclear freeze surge by citizen-activists such as Bumpers). By the end of the decade, Peace Links, as a citizen activism organization anchored in responding to the threat of nuclear weapons, declined, and Bumpers's initial passion for preventing nuclear war was overshadowed by post–nuclear freeze interests.

Certainly, Bumpers's antinuclear war ethos influenced her "post-freeze" concerns. For example, she and Peace Links continued to mentor women leaders in gatherings such as the Women for Responsible National Security Conference in Washington, D.C., in December 2000.[26] Bumpers served as a board member with the U.S. Institute of Peace, mandated as a national peace academy to provide programs, including grants, fellowships, conferences, library services, publications, and other educational activities.[27]

There is evidence that the nuclear freeze surge achieved a kind of moral success as well as some moderate policy impact. Wittner argues that organizations empowered during the 1980s peace surge were relatively successful because, rather than catering only to specific audiences such as pacifists, physicians, or women, associations such as Peace Links appealed to a broad constituency. They also, "without abandoning their sharp critique of war," intentionally appealed to mainstream America. In addition, antinuclear groups were able to mature and survive in the context of nuclear threat and unpopular wars.[28] Solo notes that it has been said about the nuclear freeze that support was "a mile wide but an inch deep."[29] While large majorities of Americans supported many of the citizen-action associations' protests against nuclear arms proliferation, support for specific details of the freeze was soft and varied widely.[30]

Cortright believes that the Cold War ended when the United States and the Soviet Union signed the 1987 Intermediate-Range Nuclear Forces Treaty, eliminating intermediate-range nuclear weapons. This action was, at least in part, the result of the 1980s antinuclear war protests. As an immediate result of the treaty, East-West relations improved dramatically, and demilitarization as well as serious discussion of limiting, if not eliminating, nuclear weapons became possible. Although the 1980s peace surge, in which Peace Links was an active participant, did not stay the development of militarism and "did not alter the core structures of the war system,"[31] the surge encouraged major policy decisions. It empowered public resistance to large-scale civil defense plans by pressing Congress to limit funding for such and pressured the administration to consider serious bargaining regarding nuclear weapons in general.[32]

Peace movements are legitimate players in foreign policy, and citizen action can be an essential force for peaceful change. Where conventional history credits the decisions of a few, usually men, in determining world events, a more inclusive perspective gives voice to the unnamed millions who participate in the great social movements that shape the course of human affairs. It recognizes the Europeans and U.S. citizens who struggled for peace and an end to the war system as the true architects of the post–Cold War era.[33]

As a significant leader in both immunization and peace advocacy, Bumpers shares the credit for public health immunization and peace movement accomplishments. Her work not only affected policy change but also helped promote education that brought valuable ideas about vaccines for children and peacemaking to the forefront. Many participants and observers of her work hold that her mentoring of women leaders in the United States and abroad remains a central contribution as well. The women leaders who grew out of the Peace Links experience continue as community activists and trailblazers in a variety of public service and professional careers. Bumpers reflects that her family and their many achievements may be her most important legacy.

In our analysis, we have discussed our interpretation of how Bumpers's underlying imagery, language patterns, and treatment of gender paradox enhanced her public and personal interactions. The prominence of Every Child By Two attests to her successes in immunization. It is one of a handful of organizations that provide solid, science-based information to the public, and it is widely recognized within the medical community. Millions of children and adults who enjoy the protection of vaccines have reason to appreciate Bumpers and the efforts of Every Child By Two. The ongoing peace organizations, including those that benefited from Peace Links and Bumpers's involvement, are also a testament to her effectiveness and energy. Women leaders in communities around the globe have reason to gratefully acknowledge Betty Bumpers's ethic of caring and mentorship.

Above all, Betty Bumpers has shown how an individual can make a difference. By seizing the chances offered by public life, she reached people across the United States and abroad. Applying her strong sense of Americana and humor, interweaving her down-to-earth use of language, she connected with many women and men who sought social justice. Beyond that, she created a meaningful personal life with an admirable and accomplished family. Her legacy in immunization, peace work, and women's leadership will continue to inspire and encourage those yet to come.

NOTES

1. Betty Bumpers, "Making Our Voices Heard," speech manuscript, WAND conference, Peace Links Records Addendum, (MC 907a), series 1, subseries 4, box 7, folder 7-10, Special Collections, University of Arkansas Libraries, Fayetteville, 1. Verb tense has been changed from present, present perfect, and future tense in the original to the past tense for citations of this speech.

2. Valerie Yow, *Recording Oral History: A Guide for the Humanities and Social Sciences*, 2nd ed. (Walnut Creek, CA: AltaMira, 2005).

3. George Lakoff, *Moral Politics: How Liberals and Conservatives Think*, 2nd ed. (Chicago: University of Chicago Press, 2002).

4. Robert Rowland, "On Mythic Criticism," *Communication Studies* 41 (1990): 101–16; Robert L. Ivie, "Metaphor and the Rhetorical Invention of Cold War 'Idealists,'" *Communication Monograph* 54 (1987): 164–82; Joyce H. Rushing, "The Rhetoric of the American Western Myth," *Communication Monographs* 50 (1983): 14–32; Colleen

Kelley and Anna Eblen, *Women Who Speak for Peace* (Lanham, MD: Rowman & Littlefield, 2002).

5. Sara Ruddick, *Maternal Thinking: Toward a Politics of Peace* (Boston: Beacon Press, 1989); Anita Taylor and Linda Perry, "Paradoxes: No Simple Matter," *Women and Language* 24 (2001): 1–6; Mari Tonn, "Militant Motherhood: Labor's Mary Harris 'Mother' Jones," *Quarterly Journal of Speech* 82 (1996): 1–21.

6. Yow, *Recording Oral History*, 229.

7. Yow, *Recording Oral History*, 229.

8. Rushing, "The Rhetoric of the American Western Myth," 15.

9. Sherry Shepler and Anne Mattina, "'The Revolt against War': Jane Addams' Rhetorical Challenge to the Patriarchy," *Communication Quarterly* 47 (1999): 153.

10. Anna Eblen and Lori Wisdom-Whitley, "Betty Bumpers's Use of Myths and Metaphors," in *Women Who Speak for Peace*, ed. Colleen Kelley and Anna Eblen (Lanham, MD: Rowman & Littlefield, 2002), 123–42.

11. Betty Bumpers, personal interview, August 2005; Bumpers's acceptance speech, National Women's Hall of Fame, October 2005.

12. Taylor and Perry, "Paradoxes," 3.

13. Taylor and Perry, "Paradoxes," 3.

14. Lakoff, *Moral Politics*, 65–107.

15. Lakoff, *Moral Politics*, 66.

16. Cathy Collins, *America's Women: 400 Years of Dolls, Drudges, Helpmates, and Heroines* (New York: HarperCollins, 2003).

17. Collins, *America's Women*, 398.

18. Lakoff, *Moral Politics*.

19. Lynn M. Stearney, "Feminism, Ecofeminism, and the Maternal Archetype: Motherhood as a Feminine Universal," *Communication Quarterly* 42 (1994): 145–59; Tonn, "Militant Motherhood," 1–21.

20. D. Lynn O'Brien Hallstein, "A Postmodern Caring: Feminist Standpoint Theories, Revisioned Caring, and Communication Ethics," *Western Journal of Communication* 63, no. 1 (1999): 32–56.

21. John Lofland, *Polite Protestors: The American Peace Movement of the 1980s* (Syracuse, NY: Syracuse University Press, 1993), 8.

22. Doug McAdam, John D. McCarthy, and Mayer N. Zald, "Social Movements," in *Handbook of Sociology* (Thousand Oaks, CA: Sage, 1988), 695–737.

23. Lofland, *Polite Protestors*, 153.

24. Lofland, *Polite Protestors*, 152.

25. Lofland, *Polite Protestors*, 213.

26. "The Good News: We, the Women Campaign," www.xmission.com/pub/lists/abolition-usa/archive/v01.n407 (accessed May 2, 2010; "Short Takes, Campaigns, Upcoming Events," www.worldpolicy.newschool.edu/wpi/projects/arms/updates/121800.htm (accessed October 14, 2012).

27. "The United States Institute of Peace," www.sourcewatch.org/index.php?title=United_States_Institute_of_Peace (accessed May 2, 2010).

28. Lawrence Wittner, "Mass U.S. Peace Organizations since 1957: SANE, the Freeze, and Peace Action" (paper presented at the International Peace Research Association Global Conference, Leuven, Belgium, July 16, 2008), 10.

29. Pam Solo, *From Protest to Policy: Beyond the Freeze to Common Security* (Cambridge, MA: Ballinger, 1988), 24.

30. David Cortright, *Peace Works: The Citizen's Role in Ending the Cold War* (Boulder, CO: Westview Press, 1993), 80.

31. Cortright, *Peace Works*, 248.

32. Cortright, *Peace Works*, 247.

33. Cortright, *Peace Works*, 2.

Bibliography

Arkansas Ties. "Cotnam History." www.arkansasties.com/Special/HistoryofWomensSuffrage.htm (accessed July 29, 2012).

"Arkansas WAND News." *WAND News Bulletin.* www.wand.org/issuesact/bbd-chapters.htm (accessed May 2, 2010).

Barnes, Paula. "Betty Flanagan Bumpers: 'An Ordinary Mother' Dedicated to Peace." In *Ordinary Women, Extraordinary Lives: Women in American History*, edited by Kriste Lindenmeyer, 247–59. Wilmington, DE: Scholarly Resources, 2000.

Brokaw, Tom. *The Greatest Generation*. New York: Random House, 1998.

Bumpers, Betty. "Article for *Unitarian Universalist World*," July 7, 1986, Peace Links Records Addendum, (MC 907a), series 1, subseries 4, box 7, folder 7-9, Special Collections, University of Arkansas Libraries, Fayetteville.

———. "I've Spent the Past Two Years" (n.d.). Peace Links Records Addendum (MC 907a), series 1, subseries 4, box 7, folder 7-9, Special Collections, University of Arkansas Libraries, Fayetteville.

———. "Making Our Voices Heard." Speech manuscript, WAND conference (n.d.). Peace Links Records Addendum (MC 907a), series 1, subseries 4, box 7, folder 7-10, Special Collections, University of Arkansas Libraries, Fayetteville.

———. "Memorable Day." Speech manuscript (n.d.). Betty Bumpers Childhood Immunization Project Papers (MC 1204), box 5, folder 2. Special Collections, University of Arkansas Libraries, Fayetteville.

———. "Remarks." Induction, National Women's Hall of Fame, Seneca Falls, New York, October 8, 2005, Special Collections, University of Arkansas Libraries, Fayetteville.

———. "Ship of State." Speech manuscript, WAND conference (n.d.). Peace Links Records Addendum (MC 907a), series 1, subseries 4, box 7, folder 7-10, Special Collections, University of Arkansas Libraries, Fayetteville.

———. "Why I Like Arkansas." Manuscript and correspondence with Bob McCord, May 6, 1986. Peace Links Records (MC 907), series 1, subseries 1, box 2, folder 2-9, Special Collections, University of Arkansas Libraries, Fayetteville.

———. "Wilton Peace Award Speech" (March 27, 1986). Peace Links Records Addendum (MC 907a), series 1, subseries 4, box 7, folder 7-9, Special Collections, University of Arkansas Libraries, Fayetteville.

Bumpers, Dale. *The Best Lawyer in a One-Lawyer Town*. Fayetteville: University of Arkansas Press, 2004.

———. Remarks, Senate proceedings. *Congressional Record*, October 1, 1982, 97–134, 513140.

Campbell, Karlyn Kohrs. "The Rhetorical Presidency: A Two-Person Career." In *Beyond the Rhetorical Presidency*, edited by Martin J. Medhurst, 179–95. College Station: Texas A&M University Press, 1996.

Carpenter, Ronald H. "America's Tragic Metaphor: Our Twentieth-Century Combatants as Frontiersmen." *Quarterly Journal of Speech* 76, no. 1 (February 1990): 1–22.

Carson, Clayborne, ed. *The Autobiography of Martin Luther King, Jr.* New York: Warner Books, 1998.

Carter, Rosalynn. *First Lady from Plains.* Boston: Houghton Mifflin, 1984.

Centers for Disease Control. "Achievements in Public Health 1900–1999: Changes in the Public Health System." www.cdc.gov/mmwr/preview/mmwrhtml/mm4850a1.htm (accessed July 20, 2012).

Centers for Disease Control and Prevention. "National Immunization Survey 2008 Table Data." www.cdc.gov/vaccines/stats-surv/nis/data/tables_2008.htm (accessed July 2010).

Collins, Cathy. *America's Women: 400 Years of Dolls, Drudges, Helpmates, and Heroines.* New York: HarperCollins, 2003.

Cortwright, Donald. *Peace Works: The Citizen's Role in Ending the Cold War*. Boulder, CO: Westview Press, 1993.

Dragonwagon, C. "I Couldn't Just Sit Around and Wring My Hands." *McCall's*, January 1983, 42–45.

Dumas, Ernie. Personal notes on transcripts of personal interview with Dale Leon Bumpers for Arkansas Governors Project, May 12, 2002, University of Arkansas, Little Rock.

Eblen, Anna, and Lori Wisdom-Whitley. "Betty Bumpers's Use of Myths and Metaphors." In *Women Who Speak for Peace*, edited by Colleen Kelley and Anna Eblen, 123–42. Lanham, MD: Rowman & Littlefield, 2002.

Encyclopedia of Arkansas. "Franklin County." http://encyclopediaofarkansas.net/encyclopedia/entrydetail.aspx?entryID=410 (accessed July 15, 2012).

"The Good News: We, the Women Campaign." www.xmission.com/pub/lists/abolition-usa/archive/v01.n407 (accessed May 2, 2010).

Goldstein, Joshua. *War and Gender: How Gender Shapes the War System and Vice Versa.* West Nyack, NY: Cambridge University Press, 2001.

Hallstein, D. Lynn O'Brien. "A Postmodern Caring: Feminist Standpoint Theories, Revisioned Caring, and Communication Ethics." *Western Journal of Communication* 63, no. 1 (1999): 32–56.

Howe, Neil, and William Strauss. *Generations: The History of America's Future 1584–2069*. New York: William Morrow, 1991.

Ivie, Robert L. "Literalizing the Metaphor of Soviet Savagery: President Truman's Plain Style." *Southern Speech Communication Journal* 51 (1986): 91–105.

———. "Metaphor and the Rhetorical Invention of Cold War 'Idealists.'" *Communication Monographs* 54 (1987): 164–82.

Kelley, Colleen. "Beyond Peace as 'Not War': The Search for a Transcendent Metaphor." *Journal for Peace and Justice Studies* 4 (1992): 54–69.

Kelley, Colleen, and Anna Eblen. *Women Who Speak for Peace*. Lanham, MD: Rowman & Littlefield, 2002.

Lakoff, George. *Moral Politics: How Liberals and Conservatives Think.* 2nd ed. Chicago: University of Chicago Press, 2002.

Lofland, John. *Polite Protestors: The American Peace Movement of the 1980s*. Syracuse, NY: Syracuse University Press, 1993.

Martin, Karen. "Portrait of a Power Woman." *Soiree* 4 (2012): 24–27.

Mayo Clinic. "Laminectomy." www.mayoclinic.com/health/laminectomy/MY00674 (accessed September 21, 2012).

McAdam, Doug, John D. McCarthy, and Mayer N. Zald. "Social Movements." In *Handbook of Sociology*, 695–737. Thousand Oaks, CA: Sage, 1988.

Mechling, E. W., and G. Auletta. "Beyond War: A Socio-Rhetorical Analysis of a New Class Revitalization Movement." *Western Journal of Speech Communication* 50 (1986): 388–404.

New School. *ATRC Updates December 18, 2000*. www.worldpolicy.newschool.edu/wpi/projects/arms/updates/121800.htm (accessed October 14, 2012).

Parry-Giles, Shawn J., and Diane M. Blair. "The Rise of the Rhetorical First Lady: Politics, Gender, Ideology, and Women's Voice, 1798–2002." *Rhetoric and Public Affairs* 5, no. 4 (Winter 2002): 565–600.

Pierson, Ruth R., ed. *Women and Peace: Theoretical, Historical and Practical Perspectives.* New York: Croom Helm, 1987.

Plotkin, Stanley A., and Walter Orenstein. *Vaccines.* 3rd ed. Philadelphia: W. B. Saunders, 1999.

Post Winery. "About Us."www.postfamilie.com/about_us.htm(accessed July 31, 2012).

Reardon, Betty A. *Sexism and the War System*. Syracuse, NY: Syracuse University Press, 1996.

Roush, Sandra W., and Trudy Murphy. "Historical Comparisons of Morbidity and Mortality for Vaccine-Preventable Diseases in the United States." *Journal of the American Medical Association* 298, no. 18 (2007): 2155–63.

Rowland, Robert C. "On Mythic Criticism." *Communication Studies* 41, no. 2 (1990): 101–16.

Ruddick, Sara. *Maternal Thinking*. Boston: Beacon Press, 1989.

Rushing, Joyce H. "The Rhetoric of the American Western Myth." *Communication Monographs* 50 (1983): 14–32.

Shepler, Sherry R., and Anne Mattina. "'The Revolt against War': Jane Addams' Rhetorical Challenge to the Patriarchy." *Communication Quarterly* 47, no. 2 (Spring 1999): 151–65.

Smith, C. Calvin. *War and Wartime Changes: The Transformation of Arkansas 1940–1945*. Fayetteville: University of Arkansas Press, 1986.

Solo, Pam. *From Protest to Policy: Beyond the Freeze to Common Security*. Cambridge, MA: Ballinger, 1988.

Stearney, Lynn M. "Feminism, Ecofeminism, and the Maternal Archetype: Motherhood as a Feminine Universal." *Communication Quarterly* 42, no. 2 (1994): 145–59.

Swerdlow, Amy. *Women Strike for Peace: Traditional Motherhood and Radical Politics in the 1960s*. Chicago: University of Chicago Press, 1993.

Taylor, Anita, and Linda Perry. "Paradoxes: No Simple Matter." *Women and Language* 24 (2001): 1–6.

Tonn, Mari. "Militant Motherhood: Labor's Mary Harris 'Mother' Jones." *Quarterly Journal of Speech* 82, no. 1 (1996): 1–21.

Totenberg, Nina. "Mrs. America for Peace." *Parade*, March 2, 1986, 16.

"The United States Institute of Peace." www.sourcewatch.org/index.php?title=United_States_Institute_of_Peace (accessed May 2, 2010).

University of Arkansas, Little Rock. "Women's Rights."Gubernatorial Papers of Dale Leon Bumpers. www.ualrexhibits.org/bumpers/?page_id=18 (accessed July 31, 2012).

"Vaccine Research Center (VRC)." www.niaid.nih.gov/about/organization/vrc/Pages/default.aspx (accessed May 4, 2010).

"Voluntary Action Center." www.handsonnetwork.org/files/resources/VCs_A_History_of_America.pdf (accessed November 13, 2010).

Wiederkehr Winery. "History." www.wiederkehrwines.com/history.html (accessed July 31, 2012).

Wittner, Lawrence, S. "Mass U.S. Peace Organizations since 1957: SANE, the Freeze, and Peace Action." Paper presented at the International Peace Research Association Global Conference, Leuven, Belgium, July 16, 2008.

Young, N. "The Peace Movement: A Comparative and Analytic Survey." *Alternative* 9 (1986): 185–217.

Yow, Valerie. *Recording Oral History: A Guide for the Humanities and Social Sciences*. 2nd ed. Walnut Creek, CA: AltaMira, 2005.

Index

Agee, Paula, 115–119
Agricultural Extension Service, 15, 16, 22, 63, 111, 146, 163
American Medical Association (AMA), 15
Ames, Iowa, 84–85, 86
Arkansas, 143–156; geography, 5, 81, 148; history of, 5–8, 13–18, 28–29, 48–50, 72, 105–111, 113. *See also specific locations*
Arkansas Art Center, 109–110; Art Mobile, 109, 110
Arkansas governor's mansion, 14–15, 18, 106–108, 111, 156, 167
Arkansas Nurses Association, 14
Arkansas Peace Links. *See* Peace Links
Arkansas River, 5, 147, 148
Arkansas Young Democrats, 38–39
Asheville, North Carolina, 43–44
Ashley, Liza, 106, 111

Baker, Joan, 156, 157–159
Balkman, Nell, 14, 15, 16, 20, 156
Bedell, Elinor, 33–34, 44
Bethesda, Maryland, xi, 131, 144–145, 147
Bond, Bill, 109–110
Bost, Dr. Roger, 115, 117
Bost, Katheryn, 115, 117
Branch, Arkansas, 55, 69, 101, 129
Bumpers, Betty: campaigning, 105–106, 122; on childrearing, 96, 101, 112–114, 149–21, 154, 166; education, first grade through high school, 55–57, 78–80; First Lady of Arkansas, xi, 3–4, 14, 22, 38, 106–118, 167; higher education, 84–87, 88, 89; marriage, 91; on personal health, 129, 165, 166; on religion, 68–69, 101–103, 153–155; on value of experience, 15, 20, 91, 113–114, 150; Senate spouse, 30, 121–135; Soviet visits, 125–127, 137, 166; work life, 81–82, 83, 91–94, 95–96; volunteerism, 27, 102–104, 147. *See also* Every Child by Two; feminism; Methodist Church; Peace Links; political wives; women and peace movement; women's rights movement; *specific Bumpers and Flanagan family members*
Bumpers, Bill (son of Betty and Dale), 96, 108, 111, 131, 151
Bumpers, Brent (son of Betty and Dale), 95–96, 111–112, 131, 144, 151
Bumpers, Brooke (daughter Betty and Dale), 107–108, 111, 131, 144, 145, 148, 150–151, 152–153; "Brooke story" in Peace Links, 27, 29, 42, 135, 137, 168; childhood illness, 98–101, 152, 167; Dale Bumpers Senate campaign, 122
Bumpers, Carroll (brother of Dale), 91, 93
Bumpers, Dale, 121–122, 125, 130; Arkansas governor, 105–119, 121; *The Best Lawyer in a One-Lawyer Town*, 6, 75, 80, 102; early years and teens, 72, 80, 83–84, 89, 156; marriage and family, 6, 23, 30, 55, 57, 91–95, 97–102, 151, 155; retirement, 130–131, 144, 145–146; U.S. Senate, 15, 18, 28, 30, 73, 117, 121–122, 125, 130
Byrd, Robert (senator), 125

Caldicott, Helen, 8
Califono, Joe, 17, 22, 133
Carson, Clayborne, xii

Carter, Jimmy, 17, 18–19, 122, 123, 125, 133
Carter, Rosalynn, 3, 17–21, 22–24, 133, 147, 167
cattle as Flanagan family business, 77–83, 84, 165; Jersey cows, 81; trading, 63, 77–78, 80, 81–83, 163
Centers for Disease Control (CDC), 13, 14, 18–19, 22, 23
Charleston, Arkansas, 6, 7, 55, 68–69; as Betty's turning point, 77–78, 79–81, 87–88; significance in Bumpers' marriage, 91, 97–102
Chernobyl, 35, 139
Chicago, Illinois, 88–89, 91–93, 106; Chicago Academy of Fine Arts, 88–89, 166; Northwestern University Law School, 72, 89, 91–93
civil rights movement, 6, 7, 8, 39; school integration in Arkansas, 7, 33, 110
Clinton, Bill, 18, 23, 49, 73, 125. *See also* Clinton, Chelsea; Clinton, Hillary; White House; William J. Clinton Presidential Library
Clinton, Chelsea, 125
Clinton, Hillary, 3, 4, 18, 35, 125, 145
Cold War, 4, 8–9, 36, 45, 135, 137, 140, 170
Committee of Soviet Women, 126–127, 137
communication and rhetoric : analysis of Betty Bumpers, xii, 3–4, 10, 161–171; social movements, 5–9, 167–171. *See also* Bumpers, Betty; civil rights movement; feminism; peace movement; social change; women's rights movement
Cortright, David, 170

Department of Health, Education, and Welfare, 17, 21, 133
Department of Health and Human Resources. *See* Department of Health, Education, and Welfare
Daschle, Laurie, 29, 35, 156
Davis, Dr. Loyal, 92–93, 123. *See also* Reagan, Nancy
Davis, Mrs., 92–93, 123. *See also* Reagan, Nancy
Denton, Jeremiah (senator), 32, 40, 157
Dumas, Ernie, 115, 116, 117–118, 119
Dust Bowl, xi, 5, 59

Eblen, Anna, xi–xii, 3–10, 161–171
Eblen, Martha Jane (Jennie), xi–xii, 42–48
Elders, Joycelyn, 16, 156
environmentalism, 46, 130, 131, 147–148
Every Child by '74, 14–17, 18, 117, 156
Every Child by Two, 17–24, 147, 171; Peet, Amanda, 24; Vaccinate Your Baby, 24

Faubus, Orval, 7, 105; governor of Arkansas, 8, 105, 106; Little Rock schools, 7
Fayetteville, Arkansas, 72, 84, 89, 116, 148
feminism, 6, 8, 9, 40, 118, 161–162, 164, 168. *See also* gender roles; women and peace movement; women's rights movement
Flanagan, Callans (brother of Betty), 55–56, 57–58, 60, 62, 81, 86, 149, 165
Flanagan, H. R. (Babe) (father of Betty), 55–56, 59–71, 77–84, 87, 89, 118, 129, 149
Flanagan, Margaret (Maggie; Mrs. Archie Schaffer) (sister of Betty), 14; childhood, 55, 57, 66; communication analysis, 165–166; teens and adulthood, 83–84, 93, 96, 97
Flanagan, Ola Callan (mother of Betty), 55–72, 77–87, 164–166; Betty's adulthood, 129; Betty's childhood, 56, 57–58, 60, 63–66, 67, 70, 72; Betty's teens, 77–78, 84, 85, 86, 87; communication analysis of influence, 164, 164–166
Flanagan, Ruth (Mrs. Lewis Wolfe) (sister of Betty): childhood, 57–58, 65–66, 71; relationship and adulthood, 91, 101, 118, 131, 149, 165–166; teens, 83, 84, 85, 86–87

Foege, William, 18, 19, 19–20, 22
Ford, Betty, 123
Ford, Gerald, 123
Forsberg, Randy, 9, 30
Fort Chaffee, Arkansas, 5, 83
Fort Smith, Arkansas, 69, 73, 98, 101, 148; as Betty's turning point, 77–87, 113
Franklin County, Arkansas, 5
Fulbright, William (Bill), 121, 122

gender roles, 6, 164–167. *See also* feminism; women's rights movement
GI Bill, 88, 91
Gorbachev, Mikhail, 126, 127
Gorbachev, Riesa, 127–128
Gordon, Jean, 115, 117
Graham, Nancy, 29
Grand Prairie, Arkansas, 55, 68, 69, 86
Gray, Bequita Bumpers (cousin of Betty and Dale), 68, 86, 87, 89, 91, 96; Dale Bumpers governor's campaign, 105–106; interview, 72–73
Great Depression, 4, 5, 55, 57, 59, 75, 77, 94, 144, 163

Hammer, Dr. Armand, 127
Harding, Deborah, 29, 126
Harriman, Pamela, 49
Hart, Gary (senator), 40
Heinz (Kerry), Teresa, 29
Hendrix College, 48
Hennie (Huhu), 96, 105, 111
human rights, 5, 6, 8. *See also* civil rights movement; women's rights movement

Iowa State University, 84–87, 114, 166

Kelley, Colleen, 3–10, 161–171

Leveritt, Mara, 38–40
Lin, Maya, 3
linguistics, 161–167
Little Rock, Arkansas, xi, 14, 48, 72–73, 106–119, 144; Old State House Museum, 106, 122; Riverfront Park, 147–148. *See also* Arkansas governor's mansion; civil rights movement; Methodist Church
Lofland, John, 8, 168–169

metaphor and imagery, 162–164, 168–169; the farm, 162–164; the mother, 164, 168–169. *See also* communication and rhetoric; myth
Methodist Church, 68–69, 80, 101–103, 108, 116, 132, 153–154; Methodist Youth Fellowship (MYF), 80, 85; Wesley, John, 132; Wesley, Susanna, 132
Miesner, Linda, 111, 115, 116, 118
Monroe, Sarah, 117
Moscow, Russia, 36, 125, 126, 137–140
Murphy, Sara, 117, 156
myth, 161–164; definition, examples of personal myth, 162–164; definition of cultural myth, 162

National Center for Voluntary Action (NCVA), 14
National Institutes of Health, 3
National League for Nursing, 14
National Peace Academy, 128, 170
National Women's Hall of Fame, xi, 3, 131
New Deal, 4, 7, 60, 163, 164
Nixon, Pat, 16, 123
Nixon, Richard, 122–123
nuclear freeze, 8–10, 30, 168–170

Obama, Barack, 17, 146
oral history, xi, 161, 165
Ozark Mountains, 5, 81, 148

Parade magazine, 4, 32, 43
Parent Teachers Association (PTA), 14, 114, 134
Passavant Hospital, 92–93, 123
Pasternak, Boris, 140–141
Peace Links: Women Against Nuclear War, 4, 4, 124, 128–129, 134–135, 137, 169–128; Arkansas Peace Links, 48, 117; Peace Child, 43, 48; Peace Day, 34, 42–44, 46–47, 48; Peace Links North Carolina (PLNC),

42–47; Peace Links Pennsylvania, 27, 45–49; Peace Links Worldwide, 44, 45, 46, 135; Peace Panel, 33, 34, 44, 134; Peace Ribbon, 31, 40; Pen Pal project, 35, 45, 135; Soviet Women's Exchange, 34–35, 40, 44–45, 126, 135, 137–138. *See also* communication and rhetoric; peace movement; political wives; women and peace movements
peace movement, U.S., 8–9, 28–47, 168–170; effects on U.S. policy, 170; history of, 8–9. *See also* communication and rhetoric; Peace Links; women and peace movement
Pisani, Amy, 20, 22–24, 147, 156
political wives: congressional wives and Peace Links, 29–30, 32, 33, 44, 49, 124, 125, 135; leadership training in Peace Links, 134; luncheon with First Lady, 124; scholarship and analysis, 6, 169. *See also* Bedell, Elinor; Carter, Rosalynn; Clinton, Hillary; Daschle, Laurie; Nixon, Pat; Reagan, Nancy; Rockefeller, Jeanette; Williams, Carol
public and private sphere, 8, 166, 167, 168, 169

Reagan, Nancy, 93, 123–124
Reagan, Ronald, 123, 124, 125
Richardson, Anne, 16
Rockefeller, Jeannette, 109–110; Arkansas Art Center, 110; art mobile, 109; governor's mansion, 107
Rockefeller, Winthrop, 105, 106, 107, 109, 148
Roosevelt, Eleanor, 4, 35
Roosevelt, Franklin Delano, 4, 63, 79; death, 86; effects of New Deal in Arkansas, 7, 79, 111; inaugural speech, 79
Rushing, Joyce, 162

Sasser, Jim (senator), 156
Sasser, Mary, 156
Schaffer, Archie (brother-in-law of Betty), 14, 84, 87
Schaffer, Archie (nephew of Betty), 115–116, 118
Schaffer, Margaret (sister of Betty). *See* Flanagan, Margaret
Schulman, Collette, 126, 138
Skuratovskaya, Larisa, 137–141
social change, 4, 6–9, 161, 167–171. *See also* communication and rhetoric
social justice, 4, 31, 46, 171
Soviet Union, 35, 44–45, 125–127, 137–141, 170
Strategic Arms Limitation Treaty (SALT I and SALT II), 9, 28

Taylor, Anita, 164
Tereshkov, Valentina, 35, 137, 139

University of Arkansas, Fayetteville Libraries Special Collections, ix, 35
U.S. Congress, 39, 40, 55, 118, 128, 131, 134, 157
U.S. Institute of Peace, 128

Vajda, Edward, 137–141
Vietnam War protests, 8
Vital Voices, 147

Walker, William (Sonny), 116, 118
Washington, D.C., 29–30, 39, 122–131
Whillock, Margaret, 48–50, 51n20
White House: Carter, 17, 18; Clinton, 49, 51n20; Nixon, 122; Obama, 146; Reagan, 40, 124
William J. Clinton Presidential Library, 147–148
Williams, Carol, 29–30, 33–35, 40, 134–135
Wittner, Lawrence, 170
Works Progress Administration (WPA), 60–61, 62. *See also* New Deal
women and peace movement, 4, 8–9, 161–171; Another Mother for Peace, 9; Women's Action for Nuclear Disarmament (WAND), 8, 30; Women's International League for Peace and Freedom (WILPF), 28, 46; Women Strike for Peace, 9. *See also* Peace Links; peace movement

women's rights movement, 6–9, 50, 140; in Arkansas, 8; Equal Rights Amendment, 8; suffrage, 7–8, 39. *See also* feminism; women and peace movement

World War II, 5–6, 7, 79, 83–88, 156, 166

About the Editors and the Contributors

Paula Agee earned her MA in communication from the University of Arkansas and her BA in psychology from Kansas University. Her scholarship and career in higher education and most recently in a Fortune 100 company has focused on relationships, oral history, communication, and transition. As a native of Arkansas and a fellow "hill woman," she has offered a unique perspective on Betty Bumpers's contribution to the people of Arkansas through her message and her relationships in this state.

Joan Baker, a retired federal employee, resides in Little Rock, Arkansas, after living in the Washington, D.C., area for more than forty years. She attended public schools in Illinois, Missouri, and Arkansas and the University of Central Arkansas in Conway. She worked on Capitol Hill for Senator Dale Bumpers and at the Pentagon for Navy JAG and volunteered in the Personal Correspondence Office at the White House in the Clinton administration. She served on the board of directors of several organizations, including Pax World, Alexandria (Virginia) Community Y, and Peace Links in Washington, D.C. (chairman of the board for two years). She and Betty Bumpers traveled extensively on behalf of Peace Links to Russia, Eastern Europe, Israel, and Japan. She is mother of two and grandmother of two.

Anna L. Eblen, professor emeritus, recently retired from Western Washington University after twenty-six years, including sixteen as department chair. Her teaching and research areas include women and social movements, peace studies, interpersonal, small group, and organization communication. Her undergraduate work was at Duke University; she received an MA from the University of West Florida and a PhD from the University of Oregon. In 2002, Colleen Kelley and Eblen coedited *Women Who Speak for Peace*, published by Rowman & Littlefield. Betty Bumpers's advocacy work has been the subject of several studies by Eblen, and the current book was inspired by Bumpers's Peace Links Worldwide and the exceptional women of Peace Links North Carolina.

Martha Jane "Jennie" Eblen received her BA in anthropology from Eckerd College, St. Petersburg, Florida, in 1976 and her MA in anthropology from the University of Tennessee, Knoxville, in 1984. She worked in the field of archaeology in western North Carolina from 1976 to 1981 and coauthored several archeological reports while working as a North Carolina archaeological assistant at Western Carolina University, Cullowhee, North Carolina. As a member of Peace Links, North Carolina, from 1985 to 1993, she worked with Betty Bumpers. She coauthored academic papers about Bumpers with her sister Anna Eblen. Currently, she lives in Asheville, North Carolina, and is a third-generation family co-owner of the Eblen Short Stop convenience stores and the Biltmore Oil Company. She serves on multiple community and state nonprofit boards and committees and has received numerous awards and honors for her volunteerism.

Colleen Kelley is an associate professor of rhetorical communication at Penn State Erie, Behrend College. She holds a PhD in rhetorical theory and criticism from the University of Oregon. She specializes in political rhetoric and has written and presented widely in peace communication studies. She coedited *Women Who Speak for Peace.* Her previous books include *Post-911 American Presidential Rhetoric: A Study of Protofascist Discourse* and *The Rhetoric of First Lady Hillary Rodham Clinton.*

Mara Leveritt is a veteran Arkansas journalist and the author of two nonfiction books. *The Boys on the Tracks* explored a series of murders set against a backdrop of drugs and prosecutor corruption. *Devil's Knot* examined the now infamous prosecution of the men known as the West Memphis Three. A feature film based on that book, starring Reese Witherspoon and Colin Firth, is due for release in 2013. Publication of her third book, *Justice Knot,* will follow. She speaks often on the inequities of the death penalty and on the need for courts to improve public confidence in the justice system by allowing live streaming of trials.

Amy Pisani is a leading authority in pediatric health advocacy. As the executive director of Every Child By Two (ECBT), Pisani has played an integral part in setting standards for childhood immunization in America today. Since 1996, she has worked with the board of directors and ECBT staff to execute the mission and goals of ECBT. She serves as a member of the Mystic, CT Rotary Club, and the National Vaccine Advisory Committee of the U.S. Department of Health and Human Services. She is a member of the board of directors of the Vaccine Education Project and the board of advisers to the Medical History Pictures Association. As a mother of two school-age children, she has firsthand experience in navigating the health care system in order to ensure timely immunization of her family. She received her MS from Gallaudet University for the Deaf and her baccalaureate degree in psychology from the Catholic University of America, Washington, D.C.

Larisa Skuratovskaya, MD, PhD, is a representative for the Russian Federation of Young Global Leadership Foundation and scientific secretary at the Institute of General Pathology and Pathophysiology, Russian Academy of the Medical Sciences. A physician who graduated from the Azerbaijan Medical Institute and the International Human Rights Center of Columbia University, New York, she researches gender, atherosclerosis, and the state of the endocrine system. She has recently studied gender aspects of public health, anthropogenic climate changes, and adaptation. Since the mid-1980s, she has taken an active part in the international women's movement, with interests in the interaction between health, the environment, and human rights. A member of the Council of International Physicians for the Prevention of Nuclear War, the Council of International Museum of Women, and the International Group on Climate Change Research of the World Council of Churches, she is also a founding member of IWF-Russia and served as president from 2001 to 2003. When Russia was the 2006 chair of the G8, she was very active in preparation and participation of the Civil Forum. Author of more than fifty publications, she also served as scientific editor of six books. She and her husband, Vadim Repin, live in Moscow, Russia.

Edward Vajda is a professor in Western Washington University's Department of Modern and Classical Languages, where he has been on the faculty since 1987. He teaches courses in Russian language, culture, and history as well as general linguistics and Inner Asian and Siberian peoples. He is currently serving as director of the Linguistics Program and recently served as director of the Center for East Asian Studies and as associate director of the Center for International Studies. He also serves as an editor of the New York–based linguistics journal *Word*. Fluent in several languages, he has authored six books and dozens of articles and reviews. His current research involves documenting the disappearing languages of Siberia. He is also affiliated with the Max Planck Institute for Evolutionary Anthropology in Leipzig, Germany, where in August 2006 he proposed the first widely accepted linguistic link between an Old World and a New World language family. He received Western Washington University's 1992 Excellence in Teaching Award and the 2011 Paul J. Olscamp Research Award.

Carol Williams is a fifth-generation Montanan. She has a BS degree in education from Western Montana College. She has had a lifetime of community activism. Her professional efforts have included teaching, assistant to the chief clerk in the Montana legislature, and a cofounder of Peace Links, an international nonprofit organization that created international exchanges for women in Russia, Eastern Europe, China, and Japan and advocated for an end to the nuclear arms race. She serves on numerous state and national boards, including Montana's Every Child By Two, and has received many awards for her efforts. She served in the 1999–2000 Montana legislature, was an unsuccessful candidate for lieutenant governor in 2000, and currently serves as a state senator from Missoula County. She has the distinction of being the first woman in Montana history to be elected by her colleagues to serve as majority (2007) and minority (2009–2013) leader. She is the wife of former Montana Congressman Pat Williams.